OCCUPATION FOR
OCCUPATIONAL THERAPISTS

OCCUPATION FOR OCCUPATIONAL THERAPISTS

Edited by

Matthew Molineux

Head of Occupational Science and Occupational Therapy
School of Health and Human Sciences
Leeds Metropolitan University, UK

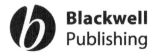

Blackwell
Publishing

© 2004 by Blackwell Publishing Ltd

Editorial offices:
Blackwell Publishing Ltd, 9600 Garsington Road, Oxford OX4 2DQ, UK
 Tel: +44 (0)1865 776868
Blackwell Publishing Inc., 350 Main Street, Malden, MA 02148-5020, USA
 Tel: +1 781 388 8250
Blackwell Publishing Asia Pty Ltd, 550 Swanston Street, Carlton, Victoria 3053, Australia
 Tel: +61 (0)3 8359 1011

First published 2004 by Blackwell Publishing Ltd

Library of Congress Cataloging-in-Publication Data

Molineux, Matthew.
Occupation for occupational therapists/Matthew Molineux.–1st ed.
 p. ; cm.
Includes bibliographical references and index.
 ISBN 1-4051-0533-X (pbk. : alk. paper)
 1. Occupational therapy.   2. Occupational therapy–Philosophy.
 [DNLM: 1. Occupational Therapy.   2. Professional Role. WB 555 M721o 2004] I. Title.

 RM735.M555 2004
 615.8′515–dc22
 2003024701

ISBN 1-4051-0533-X

A catalogue record for this title is available from the British Library

Set in 10/12.5pt Palatino
by DP Photosetting, Aylesbury, Bucks

The publisher's policy is to use permanent paper from mills that operate a sustainable forestry policy, and which has been manufactured from pulp processed using acid-free and elementary chlorine-free practices. Furthermore, the publisher ensures that the text paper and cover board used have met acceptable environmental accreditation standards.

For further information on Blackwell Publishing, visit our website:
www.blackwellpublishing.com

Dedicated to
Isabella and Holly

Contents

Preface

When I was about 15 years old, my younger sister was referred to an occupational therapist for assessment of what turned out to be perceptual motor difficulties. After hearing about what happened in her assessment and subsequent treatment I became intrigued and so investigated this profession which had previously been completely unknown to me. I read careers information, visited some occupational therapy departments, and explored the university courses offered in occupational therapy. It did not take long until I was convinced that I wanted to be an occupational therapist and so I applied in my final year of school. I was accepted and began my occupational therapy studies at The University of Queensland, Australia.

During the very first year of my undergraduate course we studied the history and philosophy of occupational therapy, with texts such as Mosey's (1981) *Occupational Therapy: Configuration of a Profession* and Cynkin's (1979) *Occupational Therapy: Toward Health Through Activities*. At the time I did not really appreciate the full complexity and power of the ideas contained in the literature I was directed towards. Furthermore, I know that in some of my early clinical work I did not pay sufficient attention to how that material should have informed my practice. Like many occupational therapists I blamed the systems in which I worked. However, over time my perspective on the practice of occupational therapy changed. Although I cannot pinpoint the exact moment at which the penny dropped, and I am sure it has been a slow process, two experiences stand out as being particularly influential.

The first was working with a client, Carol, who was referred to occupational therapy due to a head injury she had sustained in a car accident. I took over Carol's occupational therapy when her previous therapist moved jobs. After a few weeks of rolling therapeutic putty, despite her significant abilities, Carol was unhappy with her progress and generally feeling low. After a lengthy, and at times difficult, discussion Carol and I agreed to stop the therapeutic putty and make spaghetti instead. I went to her house late one afternoon and Carol made dinner for herself, her husband, her brother-in-law, and me. The change in Carol after that session was remarkable; engaging Carol in occupations and addressing her occupational needs was the key to her true recovery.

Perhaps the most powerful example of the importance of occupation to humans comes from my personal life. My maternal grandmother was an amazing woman and was so active in her home and local community that we often joked that she had a more active life than me, my sister or my parents. As she grew older her health deteriorated and ultimately her ability to do all the things she enjoyed diminished, and so she slowly and reluctantly relinquished cooking, lawn bowls, knitting, attending the horse races, playing cards with friends, and indeed most of the occupations which made her life rich and meaningful. To see her life change so significantly and the detrimental impact it had on her was a sad yet persuasive lesson in the human need for occupation.

The net result of these two experiences, along with numerous others, has resulted in my commitment to an approach to occupational therapy practice which remains true to the history and philosophy of the profession, while also incorporating more recent developments and research.

In my professional career I have been lucky to have had contact with occupational therapists who have stimulated my thinking about the profession and human occupation. These have included Susan Ryan, Anne Wilcock and Jenny Strong. Furthermore, I have worked clinically with occupational therapists who have also been committed to an occupational perspective, but more importantly have found ways to implement that in practice. From my time working with Helen Anderson and Ruth Darling, and other colleagues in Newham, I know that occupational therapists can work in ways which are consistent with their philosophy, for the ultimate benefit of their clients.

My hope for this book is that it will stimulate, encourage, and support occupational therapy clinicians and students to work in ways that are grounded in and focused on occupation. I hope you enjoy the book.

Matthew Molineux
York, UK

References

Cynkin, S. (1979) *Occupational Therapy: Toward Health Through Activities*. Boston: Little, Brown & Co.

Mosey, A.C. (1981) *Occupational Therapy: Configuration of a Profession*. New York: Raven Press.

Acknowledgements

A huge thanks to all the contributors to this book. I am grateful for your commitment to the project, and the investment of time and energy you have made to make it happen. I have enjoyed working with you and thank you for your tolerance.

To the staff at Blackwell Publishing, particularly Caroline Connelly, Lisa Whittington and Shahzia Chaudhri, I am grateful for your guidance and support in steering me through the process of producing this book. From the beginning Caroline has been enthusiastic, encouraging and accommodating, which has made the process seem so much more manageable.

Thanks to Elizabeth McKay for providing feedback on sections of the book. Your comments were honest and useful, as usual.

Finally I would like to thank Jason Ward for understanding the demands this endeavour has placed on my time, and to Peter and Marie Molineux for your never ending encouragement of all that I do.

Contributors

Editor
Matthew Molineux BOccThy, MSc, ILTM, AccOT, SROT, Head of Occupational Science and Occupational Therapy, School of Health and Human Sciences, Leeds Metropolitan University, Leeds, UK. Previously Senior Lecturer in Occupational Therapy, School of Professional Health Studies, York St John College, York, UK

Contributors
Mike Carlson PhD, Research Professor, Department of Occupational Science and Occupational Therapy, University of Southern California, Los Angeles, USA

Florence A. Clark PhD, OTR, FAOTA, Professor and Chair, Department of Occupational Science and Occupational Therapy, University of Southern California, Los Angeles, USA

Jane Cronin-Davis BA(Hons), BHSc(Hons), MSc(Crim Psych), SROT, Senior Lecturer, School of Professional Health Studies, York St John College, York, UK

Louise Farnworth BAppSci(OT), GradDipCrim, MA, PhD, AccOT, Senior Lecturer, School of Occupational Therapy, La Trobe University, Melbourne, Australia

Janet Golledge DipCOT, CertHSM, MA, SROT, Senior Lecturer, School of Professional Health Studies, York St John College, York, UK

Rachel Hayden BSc(Hons), SROT, Head Occupational Therapist, Bradgate Mental Health Unit, Leicester, UK

Clare Hocking DipOT, AdvDipOT, MHSc(OT), Principal Lecturer, School of Occupational Therapy, Auckland University of Technology, Auckland, New Zealand

Jeanne Jackson PhD, OTR, FAOTA, Associate Professor, Department of Occupational Science and Occupational Therapy, University of Southern California, Los Angeles, USA

Natasha Kerr BSc(OT), Occupational Therapist, Capital Health Region, Victoria, Canada

Amanda Lang DipCOT, BSc(Hons), MSc, Head of Occupational Therapy, Stockton Hall Hospital, York, UK

Cathy Long DipCOT, MSc, SROT, Senior Lecturer, School of Professional Health Studies, York St John College, York, UK

Joan C. Rogers PhD, OTR/L, FAOTA, Professor of Occupational Therapy, Psychiatry and Nursing, School of Health and Rehabilitation Sciences, University of Pittsburgh, Pittsburgh, USA

Gaynor Sadlo PhD, PGDipTCDHE, DipOccThy, SROT, Head of Occupational Therapy, School of Health Professions, University of Brighton, Eastbourne, UK

Karen Stagnitti BOccThy, PhD, AccOT, Senior Lecturer in Education and Training, Greater Green Triangle University Department of Rural Health, Warrnambool, Australia

Anita M. Unruh PhD, MSW, OT(C), RegNS, Professor, School of Health and Human Performance, Dalhousie University, Halifax, Canada and cross-appointed to the School of Occupational Therapy, Dalhousie University, Halifax, Canada

Joan Versnel MSc(OT), RegNS, Assistant Professor, School of Occupational Therapy, Dalhousie University, Halifax, Canada

Gail Elizabeth Whiteford BAppSc(OccTherapy), MHSc(OccTherapy), PhD, Professor and Chair of Occupational Therapy and Centre Director, Research into Professional Practice, Learning and Education (RIPPLE), Charles Sturt University, Albury, Australia

Ann A. Wilcock DipCOT, BAppScOT, GradDipPublicHealth, PhD, FCOT, Professor of Occupational Science and Therapy, Deakin University, Geelong, Australia

Jon Wright DipCOT, SROT, MSc, PGCE, ILTM, Senior Lecturer, School of Health Professions, University of Brighton, Eastbourne, UK

Sarah Yallop BAppSc(OccTh)(Hons), HIV and Sexual Health Promotion Consultant, Northern Sydney Area Health Service, Sydney, Australia

Introduction

Matthew Molineux

As outlined in the Preface, this book emerged out of my own commitment to an occupational perspective of humans and their health. My own reawakening to occupation has not been an isolated event, however, but just one example of a wider movement. This movement has been the recognition by occupational therapists, individually and collectively, that the profession must re-engage with its original vision. It is noteworthy that this movement is not a recent phenomenon, but has a long heritage in the profession. In recent times it could be suggested that the unease of therapists has grown due to changes in health and social care sectors. The pressures in these ever changing environments have meant that the scope of practice has been eroded. In some practice settings it can be seen that modern practice bears little resemblance to true occupational therapy.

Although these two conflicting forces have resulted in what seems to be a perpetual professional identity crisis, the call for a return to the profession's roots continues to survive. The desire and need to re-centre on occupation has led to important developments within the profession. These include a growing amount of research on which to base practice, and continued work to explore and develop profession specific models and approaches which focus on the occupational needs of clients. The emergence and continued growth of occupational science has been of particular significance. While the debate about the exact relationship between occupational science and occupational therapy continues, as it should, it is true to say that the new field has contributed significantly to the further development of occupational therapy knowledge and practice.

The aim of this book is to assist occupational therapy students and practitioners to reconnect with the profession's philosophy at a conceptual level, but also to see what this means for current and future practice. To that end, the book begins with a chapter which discusses the place of occupation within occupational therapy. It briefly reviews the history and development of the profession, before considering some of the dilemmas of modern practice. The book is then divided into three sections. Section one includes chapters which examine particular conceptual issues within occupational therapy, and although some may seem more theoretical than others, they all have implications for clinical practice.

The second section includes examples of how occupational therapists have worked with clients and done so within an occupational framework. It intentionally does not include examples from every field of occupational therapy practice. Rather the reader has several different examples which are likely to be useful and interesting for those working in the particular clinical fields they cover. Even for those not working in the specific settings discussed, the principles employed are likely to be relevant to many occupational therapists. Of note in this section is that while all the chapters exemplify practice which is occupationally focused, the methods utilized to achieve that end are diverse. Some chapters discuss how particular assessments and approaches to treatment enable practice to retain an occupational focus, while others highlight how an occupational science perspective is useful in achieving the same goal. In reading chapters in this section some readers may find themselves wondering how the practice presented is innovative or any different from their own practice. Those who ask this or similar questions may like to take comfort in the fact that they are not alone in working in those ways with clients. Other readers, however, may find that the practice outlined is very different from their own.

The final section includes three chapters which present a view of possible new areas of work for occupational therapists: working with people who are refugees, lifestyle redesign and public health. Given that the extent to which these approaches have been implemented varies, some of the ideas for practice are only suggestions. For this reason, readers may like to use the material presented in this section as a springboard for exploring the possibilities of future occupational therapy. All readers should be aware, however, that the issues covered in these chapters have the potential to be of use to all occupational therapists regardless of expertise or field of practice.

In using this book readers are reassured that it is not necessary to read every chapter in sequence; feel free to go directly to those that interest you first, but also explore other chapters. Finally, in order to make the most of what each chapter has to offer, it is likely that readers will wish to return to some chapters after the initial read.

Chapter 1
Occupation in Occupational Therapy: A Labour in Vain?

Matthew Molineux

1.1 Introduction

The title of this chapter is inspired by Australian penal history, in that one of the punishments used by prison officers in early Australia was called 'a labour in vain'. The precise nature of the punishment varied, but essentially it involved the prisoner engaging in a futile activity. One form of labour in vain was for prisoners to be given a metal bucket and told to polish it until the bucket shined. As the buckets were used as toilets or to clean out the prison cells there was no need for them to gleam, given that soon after the bucket had been polished it would once again be dirty: the task was futile and meaningless. At first thought, a labour in vain may seem nothing more than an interesting historical anecdote. It is my contention, however, that this early form of punishment is a useful way to consider modern occupational therapy practice. In particular, it is worth considering three key questions: do the people who receive occupational therapy as clients labour in vain, do individual occupational therapists labour in vain in their attempts to address the occupational needs of clients, and finally is the profession of occupational therapy labouring in vain in its attempts to raise awareness of the occupational needs of humans?

It is my suggestion that the answer to the first of these questions is yes, sometimes, but not always, occupational therapists do subject their clients to the clinical equivalent of a labour in vain. The answers to the remaining two questions are more complex. It is probably true that many, but not all, occupational therapists work in systems and environments which make it difficult to address the occupational needs of their clients. This is most often due to factors such as the dominance of the medical model, coupled with the significant political, institutional and financial pressures which characterize modern health and social care. The paradox, however, is that while occupational therapists are labouring to increase awareness of the occupational nature of humans, the relationship between occupation and health is becoming more widely accepted outside the profession. While it is rarely, if ever, labelled occupation, an occupational perspective is indeed on the rise.

Given the history, philosophy and growing evidence base of the occupational therapy profession, this labouring in vain is construed here as undesirable and unnecessary. In order to illustrate this, this chapter will review the place of occupation in occupational therapy, consider current occupational therapy practice in the context of this heritage and make some suggestions as to how to reduce the labouring in vain. Of course these are very complex issues and it is therefore not possible to explore them in great depth, nor to provide all the answers, and so the aim of this chapter is to highlight them and stimulate thought, and hopefully action.

1.2   Occupation in occupational therapy

At the inception of occupational therapy, the concept of occupation held centre place within the philosophy of the profession. The founders of occupational therapy based the new profession on their own personal experiences of the health enhancing effects of engagement in purposeful and meaningful activity (Peloquin, 1991a, b). George Barton, for example, had first hand experience of the health benefits of occupation. After becoming paralysed on one side of his body following surgery for gangrenous toes, Barton established Consolation House in 1914 where he, and later others, engaged in workshop activities to improve their functioning. Susan Tracey, a nurse, saw the benefits of activity when she worked with patients on surgical wards. Convinced by those early experiences, she continued to use activity with patients in a variety of settings and eventually wrote and taught others about the therapeutic use of occupation. This way of working with people with physical disabilities and psychiatric conditions became popular, and the profession grew and expanded, first in the United States of America, and then gradually around the world. Kielhofner (1992) noted that for the early part of the twentieth century there was a degree of consensus regarding the assumptions which underpinned occupational therapy practice: the essential role of occupation in human life; the link between mind and body; that lack of occupation could result in poor health and dysfunction; and conversely, that occupation could be used to restore health and function. The history of the occupational therapy profession is well documented elsewhere (see for example Peloquin, 1991a, b; Reed, 1993; Schemm, 1994; Wilcock, 1998, 2001a, 2002), and while it is beyond the scope of this chapter to trace the profession's history, one recurring issue for the profession is worth considering.

Kielhofner (1992) has noted that the 1970s saw a growing dissatisfaction among occupational therapists with the mechanistic approach that gained favour in the preceding two decades. Occupational therapists in the 1970s came to realize that human beings did not merely equal the sum of their parts. Furthermore, the approaches to treatment that the mechanistic paradigm[1] fostered were found not

---

[1] A paradigm is the 'common vision of members of a profession' (Kielhofner, 1992, p. 15).

to meet the complex needs of people with disabilities. Interestingly, there was a call for a return to the occupational roots of the profession long before the crisis in the 1970s. Reilly (1962) called for therapists in the early 1960s to demonstrate not only the occupational nature of humans, but also the ability of the profession to address the occupational needs of people.

More recently, there is still some indication that the occupational needs of people have been neglected by occupational therapists working in traditional health services. For example, Little (1993), a wheelchair user, has suggested that occupational therapists should approach their work with people with disabilities with the aim of solving everyday problems. These problems might include not just getting dressed, but also going out in public and participating in life, which might involve how to enjoy a meal at a restaurant by feeding oneself while maintaining a sense of dignity. These seem to be problems of occupational performance, which should be the focus of occupational therapists. Throughout the history of the profession occupational therapists have recognized the deficiencies of practice and called for the profession to scrutinize the occupation-health relationship and return to occupational therapy practice grounded in occupation (Reilly, 1962; Rogers, 1984; West, 1984; Yerxa *et al.*, 1989; Yerxa, 1991).

1.3   Current occupational therapy practice

From tracing the passage of the occupational therapy profession through two previous paradigms Kielhofner suggested in 1992 that occupational therapy was developing a third paradigm which incorporated the strengths of previous ones (Kielhofner, 1992). More recently Kielhofner (1997) noted that the new paradigm was again only emerging and not yet fully formed. He proposed that three broad assumptions characterize this emerging paradigm. First, is that humans have an occupational nature. Second, that humans can experience occupational dysfunction. Third, that occupation can be used as a therapeutic agent. Table 1.1 presents these assumptions along with those of previous paradigms for comparison.

From reviewing the assumptions of previous paradigms, it is clear that the emerging one is rooted firmly in the original paradigm of occupation, and yet is different. Occupation is now the dominant construct which characterizes how occupational therapists understand humans, dysfunction and intervention. This change may appear subtle, but its significance is not to be underestimated. The view now is that humans are occupational beings, not merely that occupation is an important part of human life. Similarly, rather than viewing health and ill health in terms of damage to mind and/or body, it is now conceptualized from an occupational perspective as occupational dysfunction. The idea that occupation can facilitate the restoration of function has remained in the emerging paradigm. Although the reductionist approaches which grew in popularity during the mechanist period have largely fallen out of favour, this period of the profession's history has proved valuable (Wilcock, 1991). For example, 'an important heritage from the field's second, mechanistic paradigm is the recognition of the importance of the performance components to occupation (Kielhofner, 1992, p. 54).

Table 1.1 Assumptions central to each paradigm of occupational therapy. Adapted wtih permission from Kielhofner, G. (1992). *Conceptual Foundations of Occupational Therapy.* Philadelphia: F.A. Davis.

The paradigm of occupation (1900–1950)
- Occupation plays an essential role in human life and influences health
- Occupation consists of an alternation between modes of existing, thinking, and acting
- Mind and body are inextricably linked
- Lack of occupation can result in damage to mind and body
- Occupation can be used to restore function

The mechanistic paradigm (1960s)
- The ability to perform depends on integrity of body systems
- Damage or abnormal development of body systems can result in incapacity
- Functional performance can be restored by improving or compensating for system limitations

The emerging paradigm (1980–present day)
- Humans have an occupational nature
- Humans may experience occupational dysfunction
- Occupation can be used as a therapeutic agent

The suggestion that the occupational therapy profession is in the midst of an emerging paradigm of occupation, is supported by developments within the profession. Commenting on a published review of the north American professional literature between 1900 and 1990 (McColl *et al.*, 1993), Whiteford *et al.* (2000) noted that the number of papers published which focused on occupation was initially large in the period up to 1950 (44.5% of all papers published on occupation between 1900 and 1950), this then dropped off to 19.3% between 1951 and 1980, but then increased to 36.2% in the 1981–1990 period. This is consistent with the foci of the three paradigms proposed by Kielhofner (1992) and further demonstrates that since 1980 there has been a 'resurgence of interest in occupation' (Wilcock, 1991, p. 74). The other key development has been the emergence and continued growth of occupational science. The first paper published on this topic appeared in 1989, in which it was defined as 'the study of the human as an occupational being including the need for and capacity to engage in and orchestrate daily occupations in the environment over the lifespan' (Yerxa *et al.*, 1989, p. 6). It has been suggested that one of the strengths of this new field is that it will force occupational therapists to re-engage with their philosophy and return occupation to the centre of occupational therapy (Molineux, 2000), because the focus of occupational science is humans as occupational beings (Yerxa *et al.*, 1989; Wilcock, 1993). In parallel to these developments within occupational therapy, there has been a general growing interest in occupation (although it is usually not given that name) by others outside occupational therapy (See Golledge, 1998; Wood, 1998; Molineux, 2001, 2002; for discussions of this issue).

Research from outside occupational therapy and occupational science is demonstrating the occupational nature of humans and the impact of occupation on health. For example, the Health Walks Research and Development Unit (2000) at Oxford Brookes University has been investigating the health benefits of led walks in the countryside. The original walks project was instigated by a general practitioner and since then has been developed and scrutinized. Researchers in the unit have found that in addition to the obvious impact on physical fitness, participants also reap benefits due to the social aspect of the walks, and this is consistent with the multidimensional nature of occupation (Yerxa *et al.*, 1989). The positive impact engaging in occupations has on survival has been demonstrated by a group of public health doctors in the United States of America (Glass *et al.*, 1999). This study found that although, to use their categories, social activities (e.g. attending church, playing bingo, eating out at restaurants) and productive activities (e.g. gardening, shopping, paid or unpaid work) resulted in little, if any, improvement in physical fitness, they did lower the risk of death as much as fitness activities (e.g. walking, physical exercise). While the authors of this paper did not discuss their findings in relation to the health benefits of occupation, this study supports the link between occupation and health (Molineux, 1999; Rebeiro, 1999).

This growing acceptance of the value of occupation in the lives of humans is encouraging. However, it is also somewhat problematic for occupational therapists given the way in which the profession has developed. There is much anecdotal evidence to suggest that occupational therapists, who are the alleged experts in occupation, do not understand the construct and do not address the occupational needs of their clients in practice. For example, Wood (1998) recalled a telephone call in which her sister, a business journal publisher, bemoaned the results of sending out reporters to interview occupational therapists and physiotherapists. Her sister, who had a good understanding of occupational therapy, was dismayed when the reporters returned suggesting that the professions 'were more indistinguishable than not' (Wood, 1998, p. 403). From my own experience of visiting one particular occupational therapy department, I can fully understand how the reporters could see no difference between occupational therapy and physiotherapy. I arrived at the occupational therapy department and was walking to the office to meet the student I was visiting. On my way I passed a large room and witnessed an elderly woman dressed in a flowing sari pedalling a pedal fretsaw, with no wood in sight and not even a blade in the saw.

In his book about having a stroke and undergoing rehabilitation, the author and literary editor of the *Observer* newspaper, Robert McCrum (1998, p. 139) recalled that:

> 'The part of convalescence that I found most profoundly humiliating and depressing was occupational therapy... I was reduced to playing with brightly coloured plastic letters of the alphabet, like a three year-old, and passing absurdly simple recognition tests. Sitting in my wheelchair with my Day-Glo letter blocks I could not escape reflecting on the irony of the situation. If only Milan Kundera, Kazuo Ishiguro or Mario Vargas Llosa, whose texts I had pored over with their authors, could have seen their editor at that moment.'

Similarly, Gray (1998) reported on her discussions with one man who had received occupational therapy. When asked about his experiences he recalled only that he was asked to 'pick that up there and put it over there' (p. 354). These examples focus on clients with physical disabilities, as that is my own area of clinical experience, but there are similar concerns within the field of mental health (Yau, 1995; Lloyd *et al.*, 1999). A survey of occupational therapists working in the UK in mental health conducted by Craik *et al.* (1998) demonstrated a level of role blurring. They found that 67% of their respondents felt they had carried out tasks such as giving advice about medication, testing urine for drugs and explaining blood test results. All of these accounts are powerful examples of practice which 'so heavily emphasizes performance components that it ceases to be occupational' (Gray, 1998, p. 354).

The futility of therapy which prioritises performance components over occupation has been powerfully demonstrated by Lewis (1987, p. 6) writing from a special education perspective. Lewis described an 18 year-old client, Daryl, who had been receiving a range of therapies and interventions due to an intellectual disability/learning disability. While Daryl had made progress this was of little use or relevance to him, as the excerpt below shows:

'He can sort blocks by colour, up to 10 different colours!
But, he can't sort clothes; whites from colours for washing. . .

He can roll Play Dough and make wonderful snakes!
But, he can't roll bread dough and cut out biscuits. . .

He can sit in a circle with appropriate behaviour and sing songs and play Duck, Duck, Goose.
But, nobody else in his neighbourhood his age seems to want to do that.'

One of the reasons occupational therapists find themselves in these situations is their willingness and ability to adapt to situations (Wilcock, 2001b). While this is in many ways an admirable quality, it signifies a serious deficiency in occupational therapy; practice being dictated by the individual situation rather than a professional philosophy. This was explored by Fortune (2000) when she proposed that occupational therapists working in mental health may be 'gap fillers'. In her research she presented occupational therapists with a scenario that required them to consider and describe the potential role of occupational therapy in what could be seen as a non-traditional work situation. She found that the occupational therapists described their potential role in ways that suggested they were filling a gap, and that their practice was devoid of any philosophical touchstone. Their decisions about how they might contribute in the hypothetical situation were dependent on the make-up of the team, the exact nature of the service, and were not in any way related to the occupational therapy profession. It could be that this gap filling has led to what others have called role blurring, role overlap, and role ambiguity. To rephrase Fortune (2000), it is *paradigm-independent practice* which is the cause of the mismatch between current practice and the history of the profession. While this role as gap fillers does provide occupational therapists with personal and professional identity within each work environment, it does place the profession in a very uncertain situation.

1.4   Refocusing on occupation

Working in ways that are not focused on occupation or grounded in an occupational perspective is not satisfying for individual occupational therapists, is not productive for the profession as a whole, but more importantly is not useful or meaningful for clients. Clients who experience occupational therapy like that described in the previous section are not able to reap the benefits of authentic occupational therapy. Furthermore, this is inappropriate because many clients actually want to improve their occupational performance or increase the range of occupations in which they engage, and are dissatisfied with the focus of traditional health and social care services. The solutions to the problems discussed so far are simultaneously simple and difficult. They are simple because they require occupational therapists to remember the heritage of their profession, but difficult because acting on that can be a challenge within modern work situations. All occupational therapists should, therefore, remember where they come from and, when working with clients, start where they mean to finish.

1.4.1   'Remember where you come from'

Over ten years ago, Wilcock (1991) usefully summarized the reasons why occupational therapists were not practising in ways consistent with the profession's heritage. She suggested that the construct of occupation was not fully understood by occupational therapists, probably because they have not valued the profession's philosophical base. This has resulted in 'the siphoning off of theory and philosophy from practice' (Wood, 1998, p. 404). It is, therefore, the case that many 'occupational therapists do not view the world, or work with their clients, from an occupational perspective' (Wilcock, 1991, p. 86). Instead the reductionist medical model way of viewing clients and their difficulties remains dominant in occupational therapy (Wilcock, 2000).

For some time now occupational therapy scholars have been calling for the profession to develop a philosophy which could guide education, research and practice (Reilly, 1958; Kielhofner, 1992; Yerxa, 1998; Wilcock, 1999). Wilcock (1999), drawing on earlier unpublished work of Doris Sym[2], provided strong arguments for why any profession, and in particular occupational therapy, needs a philosophy:

---

[2] Doris Sym was the founder and first principal of the Glasgow School of Occupational Therapy, Scotland, UK. In 1980 she delivered a paper at the College of Occupational Therapists' Annual Conference which explored changing professional attitudes.

- A profession based solely on skills, without a supporting philosophy, runs the risk of those skills being poached or duplicated by other professional groups, the adding and subtracting of skills when other professions change direction, or just remaining stuck in its ways.
- A philosophy would provide a common language with which occupational therapists could describe their practice. (Wilcock suggested that this might put an end to people viewing what occupational therapists do in different settings as completely unrelated.)
- A philosophy would provide a firm bedrock which future developments of the profession could be built on, and measured against, to ensure their congruence.

Although the emerging paradigm has been on the rise for some time now (Kielhofner, 1992, 1997), there is evidence to suggest that much occupational therapy practice today remains divorced from the assumptions which underpin this emerging paradigm. Although this divorce is problematic in itself, it is even more the case when one considers the growing research evidence to support an occupational view of humans, and the relationship between engagement in occupation and health (Fisher, 1998; Molineux, 2002). The reasons for this loss of occupation from occupational therapy can be identified by a review of the profession's history. Wilcock (1998) has suggested four factors: occupational therapy as prescription, the gender bias within the profession, the pursuit of professionalism and scientific reductionism.

The early influence of the medical profession over occupational therapy, like other allied health professions, meant that occupational therapy developed as a treatment that required prescription by a medical practitioner. There was very limited scope for an occupational therapist to make professional judgements about what was or was not appropriate, and in some countries that is still the case today. As Wilcock sees it, the heritage of occupational therapy as a prescribed treatment has inhibited research and development of a unique occupational perspective. The large number of women in the profession is another possible reason for the problems faced by the modern profession. Wilcock (1998, p. 190) suggests that despite early occupational therapists being proto-feminists with concerns for 'less educated or advantaged women ... they accepted subordination to medicine in a way similar to gender segregation ... of the day'. This subordination limited development of the profession as an autonomous group. There is little doubt that the alliance occupational therapy formed with medicine was beneficial for achieving greater recognition and in advancing research efforts. It is also the case, however, that while occupational therapy was dominated by medicine (e.g. requiring a prescription from a doctor in order to see a patient and having doctors in leadership positions within the professional bodies) it was virtually impossible to develop as a truly independent and autonomous profession. As discussed earlier, the mechanistic paradigm of the profession's history was one in which the link with medicine and a drive for a scientific basis resulted in a narrow focus on physical and psychological abilities. Despite the value of some knowledge and techniques developed during this period, an occupational perspective was largely lost. Some have gone so far as to suggest that this period 'was a dark age in occupational therapy's history in which occupation was figuratively lost' (Whiteford *et al.*, 2000, p. 63).

What is needed now, therefore, is for occupational therapists to re-engage with their heritage and remind themselves that they are *occupational* therapists. This will involve ensuring that clinical practice is congruent with the philosophy of the profession and the growing evidence base which exists to support it. It will require occupational therapists to articulate the uniqueness of the profession, and that is something that should not be avoided. After all, being unique is one of the hallmarks of a true profession (Reilly, 1958; Yerxa, 1967), as is the proud and vigorous use of the profession's particular media (Reilly, 1958).

The pervasive nature of occupation means that many professional groups will have some appreciation of occupation, but it is important to acknowledge that this is not to the same extent as occupational therapists. The occupational paradigm is what should bind all occupational therapists together. Although the precise ways in which therapists work might differ according to the particular models and approaches employed, all should be taking an occupational perspective. Making this change will mean the profession is no longer merely a gap filler, and that occupational therapists can rest easy knowing that practice is paradigm-dependent, and enjoy the sense of identity and role that brings. More importantly, however, occupational therapists can take comfort in knowing that the skills and knowledge of the profession are being used to maximal effect for clients.

1.4.2   'Start where you mean to finish'

While an occupational perspective is not new to occupational therapists, although many may have lost sight of it, the real challenge in the modern world is acting on that perspective. Because the remainder of this book includes many examples of how occupational therapists can, and do, practise in ways consistent with the professional philosophy, this will not be given great attention here. Before highlighting some ways in which implementing an occupational perspective in practice can be facilitated, one point is worth making. When confronted with a barrier to working in an occupational way with clients, occupational therapists must reflect on the situation and determine whether or not the barrier is real or merely perceived. While this may seem self-evident, I would argue that sometimes occupational therapists fail to overcome barriers because they make an inaccurate assessment of the nature of the barrier. A real barrier is one that is not amenable to change within the jurisdiction of the occupational therapist, the occupational therapy service (e.g. in a clinical setting) or the occupational therapy profession. A perceived barrier, on the other hand, is one that seems fixed, but on closer inspection and perhaps with slightly greater personal investment, is actually something that can be overcome. It is also important to remember that when seeking to implement occupational interventions seemingly small changes can pay large dividends.

The first aspect of 'starting where you mean to finish' is to recognize that occupational therapists view humans and health differently from other professional groups. Rogers (1982) documented that occupational therapists are, by definition, more concerned with the occupational implications of disease than the disease itself. For example, disorder has traditionally been viewed within the medical model in terms of irregularity in the function and/or structure of the human body. Although this is changing, demonstrated by the *International Classification of Functioning and Disability* (World Health Organization, 2001), it is fair to say that many current health care systems remain dominated by this perspective. In contrast, occupational therapy views disorder as dysfunction in occupational performance which results 'in an inability to effectively accomplish daily tasks and to enact occupational roles' (Rogers, 1982, p. 31). Given that the focus is on occupational performance, it could be suggested that the precise pathology which has resulted in dysfunction is of little relevance to occupational therapists. Of course, this is not entirely true, but it is important that occupational therapists understand the relative importance of the two different constructs to their practice. The relationship between, and relative importance of, pathology and occupational performance have been documented in the professional literature. For example, in the clinical reasoning research conducted by Mattingly and Fleming (Fleming, 1991; Mattingly, 1991a, b; Mattingly & Fleming, 1994), while occupational therapists were found to be interested in the pathology of the client's condition, they were more concerned with how the individual experienced the condition. This issue has been incorporated into professional documents and frameworks which guide practice (see, for example, Canadian Association of Occupational Therapists, 1991; American Occupational Therapy Association, 1994, 2002), but two particular contributions to the professional knowledge base will be outlined very briefly.

The occupational diagnosis is a useful way of understanding client difficulties in occupational performance and it makes the relationship between occupational performance and underlying pathology explicit (Rogers & Holm, 1989; Rogers in Chapter 2). An occupational diagnosis is a statement that describes the way in which disease, disability, or any other factor, impacts on occupational performance (Rogers & Holm, 1989). As such, while not ignoring the underlying pathology, it gives primacy to the implications for occupational performance. This is discussed in more depth in the next chapter, but briefly the occupational diagnosis comprises four elements. First, is the descriptive element which describes the functional problem faced by the client. Second, is the explanatory component which describes the aetiology of the functional problem. Third, are the signs and symptoms which have provided the cues for the occupational therapist, and resulted in his/her ability to propose the aetiology of the difficulty. Finally, is the pathology which is the particular medical or psychiatric problem which underlies the functional problem and gives rise to the signs and symptoms. Even from this brief overview it is possible to see how conceptualizing client difficulties in this way requires the occupational therapist to focus first and foremost on the client's occupational performance difficulties.

The other useful way of ensuring a focus on occupation in clinical practice is to ensure that assessments are occupationally focused. Hocking (2001) usefully proposed a framework for implementing occupation-based assessment, which demonstrates the relative importance of performance component deficits. The first task of assessment, in her framework, is to understand the client as an occupational being, that is, to understand 'the meanings [clients] experience and express through occupation' (p. 464). Next, is to understand the function those occupations serve in the context of the client's daily life, overall lifestyle, and even how those occupations impact on other individuals. The third stage requires the occupational therapist to gain an understanding of the form of the particular occupation in question, by attending to 'the nature and extent of any observable disruption to performance and identifying occupational performance skills and environmental opportunities that support performance' (p. 465). It is only at this stage in the process that the occupational therapist begins to examine (in detail) deficits in occupational performance components. The strength of this framework is that it places understanding the client as a unique occupational being at the start of the assessment process. In doing so it delays attention to performance components until it can be used effectively within a wider occupational perspective.

The key to 'starting where you mean to finish' lies in the focus of the assessment stage of the occupational therapy process. Given that assessment guides subsequent treatment planning and implementation, it is important to ensure that assessment focuses on what occupational therapists can and should be helping clients to address: problems with performing and managing occupations. After all, 'therapists who focus their evaluations solely on performance components risk focusing treatment around those components, thus failing to address critical occupational issues'. (Hocking, 2001, p. 463)

1.5   Conclusion

This chapter has proposed that aspects of modern occupational therapy practice may be likened to the early Australian prison punishment, a labour in vain. From a review of some of the literature which has examined and critiqued current clinic practice it seems that there may be some substance in this assertion. Paradoxically, there are developments within and outside the profession which mean that it is probably possible to minimize, if not completely eliminate, the need for occupational therapists and, more importantly, our clients, to labour in vain. The occupational therapy profession is founded on a sound philosophy which is now supported by a growing evidence base. Most exciting, is that some of the evidence is being generated outside occupational therapy and so it is clear that an occupational perspective is gaining acceptance. Two maxims for occupational therapy practitioners have been proposed: 'remember where you are coming from' and 'start where you mean to finish'. Practice guided by these principles will be based on the professional philosophy of occupation and health, and will focus from the outset on the occupational needs of our clients. While it is recognized that working in an occupationally focused manner is challenging in many health and social care environments of today, it is also recognized that not working in that way is to deny our clients the full benefits of occupational therapy. Let future occupational therapy labours not be in vain and our clients' experiences of occupational therapy be meaningful and relevant to their everyday lives.

References

American Occupational Therapy Association (1994). Uniform terminology for occupational therapy. *American Journal of Occupational Therapy, 48* (11), 1047–1054.

American Occupational Therapy Association (2002). Occupational therapy practice framework: domain and process. *American Journal of Occupational Therapy, 56* (6), 609–639.

Canadian Association of Occupational Therapists (1991). *Occupational Therapy Guidelines for Client-centered Practice*. Toronto: CAOT Publications.

Craik, C., Chacksfield, J. & Richards, G. (1998). A survey of occupational therapy practitioners in mental health. *British Journal of Occupational Therapy, 61* (5), 227–234.

Fisher, A. (1998). Uniting practice and theory in an occupational framework. *American Journal of Occupational Therapy, 52* (7), 509–521.

Fleming, M. (1991). The therapist with the three-track mind. *American Journal of Occupational Therapy, 45* (11), 1007–1014.

Fortune, T. (2000). Occupational therapists: is our therapy truly occupational or are we merely filling gaps? *British Journal of Occupational Therapy, 63* (5), 225–230.

Glass, T., De Leon, C., Marottoli, R. & Berkman, L. (1999). Population based study of social and productive activities as predictors of survival among elderly Americans. *British Medical Journal, 319*, 478–483.

Golledge, J. (1998). Is there unnecessary duplication of skills between occupational therapists and physiotherapists? *British Journal of Occupational Therapy, 61* (4), 161–162.

Gray, J. (1998). Putting occupation into practice: occupation as ends, occupation as means. *American Journal of Occupational Therapy, 52* (5), 354–364.

Health Walks Research and Development Unit (2000). *Proceedings: Health Walks Research and Development Unit Symposium*. Oxford: Oxford Brookes University.

Hocking, C. (2001). Implementing occupation-based assessment. *American Journal of Occupational Therapy, 55* (4), 463–469.

Kielhofner, G. (1992). *Conceptual Foundations of Occupational Therapy*, 1st edn. Philadelphia: F.A. Davis.

Kielhofner, G. (1997). *Conceptual Foundations of Occupational Therapy*, 2nd edn. Philadelphia: F.A. Davis.

Lewis, P. (1987). A case for teaching functional skills. *TASH Newsletter, 13* (12), 6.

Little, J. (1993). The fine line. *American Journal of Occupational Therapy, 47* (11), 1048–1049.

Lloyd, C., Kanowski, H. & Maas, F. (1999). Occupational therapy in mental health: challenges and opportunities. *Occupational Therapy International, 6* (2), 110–125.

McColl, M., Law, M. & Stewart, D. (1993). *Theoretical Basis of Occupational Therapy: an Annotated Bibliography of Applied Theory in the Professional Literature*. Thorofare: Slack.

McCrum, R. (1998). *My year off*. London: Picador.

Mattingly, C. (1991a). The narrative nature of clinical reasoning. *American Journal of Occupational Therapy, 45* (11), 998–1005.

Mattingly, C. (1991b). What is clinical reasoning? *American Journal of Occupational Therapy,* 45 (11), 979–986.

Mattingly, C. & Fleming, M. (1994). *Clinical Reasoning: Forms of Inquiry in a Therapeutic Practice.* Philadelphia: F.A. Davis.

Molineux, M. (1999). Activity and occupation (Letter). *British Medical Journal, 319.* Retrieved 24 August 1999, from http://www.bmj.com/cgi/eletters/319/7208/478#4371

Molineux, M. (2000). Another step in the right direction (Editorial). *British Journal of Occupational Therapy, 63* (5), 191.

Molineux, M. (2001). Occupation: the two sides of popularity. *Australian Occupational Therapy Journal, 48,* 92–95.

Molineux, M. (2002). The age of occupation: an opportunity to be seized. *Mental Health OT, 7* (1), 12–14.

Peloquin, S. (1991a). Occupational therapy service: individual and collective understandings of the founders, Part 1. *American Journal of Occupational Therapy, 45* (4), 352–360.

Peloquin, S. (1991b). Occupational therapy service: individual and collective understandings of the founders, Part 2. *American Journal of Occupational Therapy, 45* (8), 733–744.

Rebeiro, K. (1999). In support of meaningful occupation for the elderly (Letter). *British Medical Journal, 319.* Retrieved 26 August, 1999 from http://bmj.com/cgi/eletters/319/7208/478#4395

Reed, K. (1993). The beginnings of occupational therapy. In: H. Hopkins and H. Smith (Eds), *Willard and Spackman's Occupational Therapy* (pp. 26–43). Philadelphia: J.B. Lippincott.

Reilly, M. (1958). An occupational therapy curriculum for 1965. *American Journal of Occupational Therapy, 12* (6), 293–299.

Reilly, M. (1962). Occupational therapy can be one of the great ideas of twentieth century medicine. *American Journal of Occupational Therapy, 16* (1), 1–9.

Rogers, J. (1982). Order and disorder in medicine and occupational therapy. *American Journal of Occupational Therapy, 36* (1), 29–35.

Rogers, J. (1984). Why study human occupation? *American Journal of Occupational Therapy, 38* (1), 47–49.

Rogers, J. & Holm, M. (1989). The therapist's thinking behind functional assessment, Part I. In: C.B. Royeen (Ed.), *AOTA self study series: Assessing Function.* Rockville, Md.: American Occupational Therapy Association.

Schemm, R. (1994). Bridging conflicting ideologies: the origins of American and British occupational therapy. *American Journal of Occupational Therapy, 48* (11), 1082–1088.

West, W. (1984). A reaffirmed philosophy and practice of occupational therapy for the 1980s. *American Journal of Occupational Therapy, 38* (1), 15–23.

Whiteford, G., Townsend, E. & Hocking, C. (2000). Reflections on a renaissance of occupation. *Canadian Journal of Occupational Therapy, 67* (1), 61–69.

Wilcock, A. (1991). We are what we do: an occupational perspective on life, health and the profession. In: *Proceedings of the Australian Association of Occupational Therapists Conference 1991* (pp. 73–93). Adelaide: Australian Association of Occupational Therapists.

Wilcock, A. (1993). A theory of the human need for occupation. *Journal of Occupational Science: Australia, 1* (1), 17–24.

Wilcock, A. (1998). *An Occupational Perspective of Health.* Thorofare, NJ: Slack.

Wilcock, A. (1999). The Doris Sym Memorial Lecture: developing a philosophy of occupation for health. *British Journal of Occupational Therapy, 62* (5), 192–198.

Wilcock, A. (2000). Development of a personal, professional and educational occupational philosophy: an Australian perspective. *Occupational Therapy International, 7* (2), 79–86.

Wilcock, A. (2001a). *Occupation for Health. Volume 1: A Journey from Self Health to Prescription.* London: College of Occupational Therapists.

Wilcock, A. (2001b). Occupational science: the key to broadening horizons. *British Journal of Occupational Therapy, 64* (8), 412–417.

Wilcock, A. (2002). *Occupation for Health. Volume 2: A journey from Prescription to Self Health.* London: College of Occupational Therapists.

Wood, W. (1998). It is jump time for occupational therapy. *American Journal of Occupational Therapy, 52* (6), 403–411.

World Health Organization (2001). *International Classification of Functioning and Disability: ICF.* Geneva: World Health Organization.

Yau, M. (1995). Occupational therapy in community mental health: do we have a unique role in the interdisciplinary environment? *Australian Occupational Therapy Journal, 42* (3), 129–132.

Yerxa, E. (1967). Authentic occupational therapy. *American Journal of Occupational Therapy, 21* (1), 1–9.

Yerxa, E. (1991). Occupational therapy: an endangered species or an academic discipline in the twenty-first century? *American Journal of Occupational Therapy, 45* (8), 680–685.

Yerxa, E. (1998). Occupation: the keystone of a curriculum for a self-defined profession. *American Journal of Occupational Therapy, 52* (5), 365–372.

Yerxa, E., Clark, F., Jackson, J., Parham, D., Pierce, D., Stein, C. & Zemke, R. (1989). An introduction to occupational science, a foundation for occupational therapy in the twenty-first century. *Occupational Therapy in Health Care, 6* (4), 1–17.

Section A
Exploring the Nature of Occupation

Chapter 2
Occupational Diagnosis

Joan C. Rogers

2.1 Introduction

Occupational diagnosis refers to both the cognitive processes used by the occupational therapy practitioner to formulate a statement summarizing the client's occupational status, and the outcome of that process, the diagnostic statement. This chapter begins by charting the conceptual and empirical milestones surrounding occupational diagnosis and diagnostic reasoning. Next, in the section relating the occupational diagnosis to occupational therapy and occupational science, the benefits of a uniform nomenclature and a classification system are discussed. The pivotal role of the occupational diagnosis for occupation-based practice is then argued. Lastly, several suggestions are made for research relating problem formulation to expected outcomes to explicate diagnostic reasoning.

2.2 Overview of the literature

2.2.1 Conceptual developments

In 1960, Reilly challenged occupational therapists to 'search out and identify the thinking process we use to solve our clinical problems.' She characterized our thinking as having emerged from the 'all-inclusive generalization' stage, where activity was health promoting for all occupational therapy clients to the 'standard operating procedure' stage, where structured routines were devised for specific pathologies. Reilly's challenge to develop a scientific mode of thinking was embraced by Line (1969), who proposed adopting the case method. The case method is a problem-solving process that fosters the application of knowledge for defining and resolving problems. Data are collected, classified, analysed and interpreted in accordance with a clinical frame of reference and transformed into a definition of the problem and subsequently an action plan.

Although Day (1973) articulated the relationship between cause identification and problem identification, there was little development of either the concept of diagnostic reasoning or diagnosis in occupational therapy, until Rogers' qualitative study of practitioners (Rogers & Masagatani, 1982) and her Eleanor Clarke Slagle Lectureship (1983). The term, occupational therapy diagnosis, was introduced to refer to the concise summary of a client's disruptions in occupational role that are amenable to occupational therapy. Rogers viewed diagnostic decisions as guided by clinical questions. One major question, 'what is the client's occupational profile?' contained two subquestions: 'what are the client's strengths or abilities?' and 'what are the client's deficits or needs (occupational therapy diagnosis)?'

Hence, the occupational diagnosis, which targets the deficit to be treated by the occupational therapist, was viewed as only one outcome of diagnosis. Because the endpoint of diagnosis provides the starting point for intervention, it needs to consider all information required for intervention planning. Knowing what clients can do informs the planning process as much as knowing what they cannot do, because strengths can be used to compensate for deficits. Hence, the occupational profile, by summarizing the positive and negative aspects of performance, provides the cues needed for intervention planning. The occupational diagnosis, however, is a pivotal concept because it summarizes the need for occupational therapy and identifies the entity for which occupational therapists can be held professionally accountable.

Occupational diagnosis

Rogers and Holm (1989) advanced the concept of the occupational therapy diagnosis by suggesting a structure for practitioners to use to summarize their diagnostic reasoning. The occupational therapy diagnostic statement consists of four components: descriptive, explanatory, cue and pathological.

The *descriptive component* identifies the problem(s) that are amenable to occupational therapy. It names task disabilities, such as difficulty dressing, or social role dysfunctions, such as difficulty working as a seamstress. A task disability occurs at the level of individual tasks, while a social role dysfunction occurs at the level of social role, which is comprised of many tasks.

The *explanatory component* indicates the practitioner's hypothesis about the most likely cause or aetiology of the problem or social role dysfunction. A dressing disability, for example, might be caused by: sensory impairment (e.g. low vision, paraesthesia); physical impairment (e.g. limited movement or strength); cognitive impairment (e.g. apraxia, amnesia); affective impairment (e.g. lack of motivation, fear of injury); physical contextual hindrance (e.g. architectural barrier); or social contextual hindrance (e.g. restrictive attitude of caregiver). More than one cause of a problem may be listed in the diagnostic statement. The explanatory component is critical for planning intervention because the plausibility of solutions differs based on aetiology. For example, a dressing disability secondary to limited range of movement might be managed through self-help devices, clothing modifications or adaptive dressing techniques, while one due to a short-term memory deficit would require external prompting by an automated device or a personal care attendant.

The *cue component* indicates the cues that led the practitioner to recognize the problem and its aetiology. Cues may be symptoms or signs. Symptoms of a problem are the subjective data provided by the client and/or the client's family members or caregivers. A client may report, for example, that 'I am unable to comb my hair' or 'I cannot hold my secretarial position because I can no longer type'. Comments such as these direct the practitioner's attention to specific task disabilities. Although clients can target specific tasks, it is considerably more difficult for them to delineate the cause of the problem, although this is sometimes possible. For instance, a client may say, 'I am unable to comb my hair because I cannot reach the back of my head' or 'I can no longer type because my arthritic fingers no longer hit the right keys'. Obviously, the latter statements are more insightful than the former statements and provide more cogent direction for the collection of signs. Signs of problems are the objective data collected by the practitioner through the evaluative tools of occupational therapy. To gather objective data about an impairment in reaching, the practitioner would be likely to do an active range of movement test, while a typing disability would be observed in the actual or simulated work setting.

The *pathological component* specifies the medical (e.g. rheumatoid arthritis, macular degeneration) or psychiatric (e.g. depression, dementia) pathology that underlies the problem. Pathology is treated by physicians through medication, surgery, or psychotherapy. The nature of the pathology, the prognosis and pathology-related contraindications establish parameters for occupational therapy interventions. A deficit in meal preparation would be treated differently, in occupational therapy, if the underlying cause was an irreversible condition such as chronic obstructive pulmonary disease compared to a potentially curable one such as depression.

The *occupational therapy diagnostic statement* thus consists of the descriptive (functional problem) + explanatory (etiology of the problem) + cue (signs and symptoms) + pathological (medical or psychiatric basis) components. An occupational therapy diagnosis might state, Mrs Bright is unable to prepare meals for herself (description) related to a memory deficit (explanatory) as evidenced by her: repeated requests for instructions; inability to remember salting the soup; failure to remove the soup when it boiled; and burning the corner of the pot holder (cues); caused by dementia of the Alzheimer type (pathological).

Reasoning yielding the occupational therapy diagnosis

To describe the reasoning process leading to the occupational diagnosis, Rogers and Holm (Rogers, 1983; Holm & Rogers, 1989; Rogers & Holm 1989, 1991) proposed casting the diagnostician as a data collector, organizer, selector, and interpreter (Elstein *et al.*, 1978). By collecting, organizing, selecting and interpreting data, practitioners create an image of the client. From the time practitioners receive a referral and read words, such as stroke, hemiplegia, or depression, they begin to develop an idea of the client's problems and strengths. Newell & Simon (1972) refer to this image as a problem space. As practitioners interact with clients and evaluate their performance, this image becomes more refined. Occupational therapy knowledge stored in memory and that known tacitly through experience is combined with new data about the client. When clients' problems closely match those expected from memory and experience, thinking is automatic but mindful. However, when new data deviate markedly from the expected clinical image, more active problem solving takes place to generate a clinical image that more accurately reflects the client's status.

Active problem formulation requires the collection of data to describe the problem and identify its cause(s). From the abundance of data collected, practitioners select the data that are most relevant to the problems under consideration. Data that have diagnostic value are called cues. Because humans have limited capacity for storing data in short-term memory, early in the diagnostic process practitioners begin to organize the data that they are collecting. A primary strategy for organizing data is developing hypotheses about why performance is limited. Cues take on meaning in the context of hypotheses and are easier to remember when organized in this way.

One or more hypotheses may be developed to explain a problem. In observing a client perform bath transfers, the practitioner might hypothesize that the client lacks sufficient lower limb strength as evidenced by the following cues: she plopped down to the bottom of the bath, she pulled herself up from the bottom of the bath by using the soap dish. Additionally, the practitioner might hypothesize that the problem in executing bath transfers was apraxia secondary to cognitive impairment. Cues supporting this interpretation might be the client's attempts to rise from the bath through rocking with her feet straight out in front of her and her resistance to getting into the bath 'because I won't be able to get out'. Once a hypothesis is formulated, cue collection becomes very focused with the intent of confirming or disconfirming it. For example, a manual muscle test might be done to confirm a deficit in lower limb strength. At some point in the diagnostic process, the most plausible hypothesis is selected to serve as the starting point for intervention.

Mattingly (1991) argued against the scientific method, with its emphasis on hypothesis testing, cause and effect relationships, and generalization, as an appropriate mode of clinical reasoning for occupational therapy. Instead, she advocated narrative reasoning in which practitioners think with stories to understand the meaning of disability to clients. Using data from the same study as Mattingly, Fleming (1991a) expanded the clinical reasoning repertoire to include: procedural reasoning for physical performance problems; interactive reasoning for understanding clients as individuals; and conditional reasoning for integrating procedural and interactive reasoning and predicting potential changes in performance post-intervention. Schell & Cervero (1993) added a fifth option, pragmatic reasoning, to take into account the influence of contextual factors, such as reimbursement and equipment availability. Roberts (1996) countered this proliferation of reasoning models in occupational therapy by arguing these variant modes of reasoning might preferably be conceptualized as the same reasoning method applied to different content.

2.2.2   Empirical studies

The impetus for Rogers' Slagle lecture was her study of practitioners' reasoning during the initial evaluation of clients with physical impairments in an acute care setting (Rogers & Masagatani, 1982). The findings indicated that in the majority of problem statements the descriptive components were physical impairments and the explanatory components were medical pathologies. However, when the descriptive component identified an activity limitation, such as a dressing dis-ability, the explanation was formulated as an impairment, which in turn was attributed to a medical pathology. Except for the absence of the cue component, this line of reasoning is consonant with the format outlined above for the occu-pational diagnosis. The pilot study revealed that practitioners' problem state-ments were heavily influenced by medical diagnoses, which were used to generate a standard problem list. The list was revised using cues collected during the evaluation. Practitioners used few cues to identify problems and had con-siderable difficulty distinguishing normal from abnormal cues. For example, they were reluctant to state the range of normalcy encompassed by 'within normal limits' and 'functional'. For activity limitations, practitioners often refrained from diagnosing problems that could be readily resolved, by exchanging activity materials or using contextual resources. Thus, a client's inability to tie shoes was discounted because slip-on shoes could be worn or a caregiver could tie them.

Barris (1987) conducted a study similar to that of Rogers & Masagatani (1982) with practitioners working in mental health. From the data presented, a clear picture of problem formulation does not emerge. However, in contrast to prac-titioners working in physical disabilities, when gathering data, these practitioners were reluctant to consult a client's medical record before meeting the client because of concerns about bias. They assessed behaviours in more depth. As with their counterparts in physical rehabilitation, who devised problem lists from patients' medical diagnoses, a standard operating mode of thinking was apparent in their use of departmentally formulated assessments and goal checklists.

Hagedorn (1996) confined her investigation to the first decision experienced practitioners made about common physical performance problems. She described practitioners' reasoning as schematic processing. When practitioners were con-fronted with a particular condition, the dysfunction schema for this condition came automatically to mind. The schema contained the knowledge and experience that practitioners had of this condition. It enabled automatic processing of information and rapid decision making. The occupational therapy process was employed in a 'free and unstructured fashion', meaning that reasoning jumped to and from problem identification, goal setting, intervention planning, prediction and addi-tional data collection. Once problems were recognized, so were the solutions.

The Clinical Reasoning Study initiated in 1986 by the American Occupational Therapy Foundation and the American Occupational Therapy Association

(AOTA) had as a primary aim describing practitioners' clinical reasoning processes, inclusive of intervention (Gillette & Mattingly, 1987). Of the various types of reasoning identified (narrative, procedural, interactive and conditional), diagnosis falls under procedural reasoning. As described by Fleming (1991b) the problem-solving methods used by physicians to diagnosis disease, prognosticate about its course and prescribe treatment, were evidenced in the reasoning of experienced practitioners to identify problems, set goals, and plan treatment. In addition to the analytical processes involved in cue identification and interpretation, and hypothesis generation and evaluation, practitioners employed reasoning modes rooted in tacit (non-linguistic) knowledge, such as recognizing a problem, recognizing aspects of a problem and affirming that a problem was representative of a set of problems.

Following the tradition of the Clinical Reasoning Study, several studies examined practitioners' reliance on different reasoning modes and novice-expert differences in reasoning. Thus, Munroe (1996) found that community based practitioners were more apt to describe strategies involving decision making and reflection rather than reasoning, but that the latter could be elicited through interview. Using a case analysis, Medhurst and Ryan (1996) found that procedural strategies were employed throughout a session. Compared to novices, experts exhibited more narrative and conditional reasoning (McKay & Ryan, 1995) and valued clinical reasoning factors supported by scientific and narrative reasoning more highly (Strong *et al.*, 1995). In addition, experts' problem formulations were qualitatively but not quantitatively different (Robertson, 1996).

Neistadt (1987) explored the critical issue of teaching clinical reasoning to entry-level students. Following meetings with people with physical disabilities, students were required to construct problem, goal and plan lists specific to the speaker, under time limited conditions. Over one semester, significant improvement was detected in the students' diagnostic and treatment planning skills and about one-third of the students designated the course as one of the most helpful in preparing them for practice. Slater and Cohn (1991) proposed a similar educational programme for practitioners, but they did not test the model.

2.3   Occupational diagnosis in occupational science and occupational therapy

Although the occupational diagnosis is recognized as a pivotal concept linking evaluation and intervention, our profession has no agreed upon structure for devising diagnostic statements, no common labels for these statements, and no taxonomy for organizing them. In discussing the significance of problem formulation, Parham (1987, p. 557) commented, 'In problem setting, the therapist names what will be attended to in practice, and frames the context for intervention.' Naming or labelling concepts is the most elementary level of theory building (Dickoff & James, 1975) because concepts (labels + definitions) are the building blocks of theory. By naming concepts, theory provides a language for the 'what' of occupational therapy. By relating one concept to another, theory provides a logic for occupational therapy. It organizes concepts so as to explain occupation and occupational dysfunction.

The lack of a universally accepted nomenclature for disability has clinical as well as theoretical significance. This may be appreciated by comparing the labels and definitions of the same task using several systems. For illustrative purposes, the definitions of the concept 'washing the body' from the *International Classification of Functioning, Disability and Health* (ICF) of the World Health Organization (WHO, 2001), the *Occupational Therapy Practice Framework* (Framework) of the AOTA (2002), the *Uniform Data System for Medical Rehabilitation* (1996) as portrayed on the Functional Independence Measure (FIM^{TM}), and the commonly used Barthel Index (Mahoney & Barthel, 1965) were compared. As is evident from Table 2.1, the task of washing the body may be labelled washing oneself (ICF), bathing, showering (Framework), bathing self (Barthel Index) or bathing (FIM^{TM}) and none of the definitions are identical. Accordingly, Ms Trium, who can bathe herself, except for her back, but is unable to transfer independently into the bath or shower would have a disability based on the ICF, the Framework, and the Barthel Index, but not on the FIM^{TM}. From a theoretical perspective, although theoreticians and researchers define the meaning of concepts in the context of their own studies, the failure to abide by a uniform terminology makes it difficult to compare the findings of one study, using one meaning of a disability, with a second study, using another definition of disability. Hence, the research that is needed to guide practice accumulates slowly. From a clinical standpoint, when the number of disabilities in daily living activities is used to qualify individuals for health care services, such as for Medicare benefits in the United States, differences in the way in which activities are defined can have negative consequences for clients.

Table 2.1   Cleaning the body.

ICF: Washing oneself
Washing and drying one's whole body, or body parts, using water and appropriate cleaning and drying materials or method, such as bathing, showering, washing hands and feet, face and hair, and drying with a towel.
Inclusions: washing body parts, the whole body, and drying oneself.
Exclusions: caring for body parts, toileting.

AOTA (2002): Bathing, showering
Obtaining and using supplies, soaping, rinsing and drying body parts, maintaining bathing positions, and transferring to and from bathing positions.

Barthel Index: Bathing self
Patient may use a bath, a shower or take a complete sponge bath. He or she must be able to do all steps involved in whichever method is employed without another person being present.

Functional Independence Measure (FIM^{TM}): Bathing
Includes bathing (washing, rinsing and drying) the body from the neck down (excluding the neck and back). May be either bath, shower, or sponge/bed bath. Performs safely.

Since the format of the occupational therapy diagnostic statement was first proposed by Rogers & Holm (1989), there has been no further development of the concept of the occupational therapy diagnosis and occupational therapists continue to have no consensus about how to articulate what they treat. Beginning in 1979 and continuing to the fourth revision in 2002, the AOTA spearheaded efforts to identify and define the core concepts of occupational therapy. Although the original impetus for uniform terminology came from the federal government, in response to a need to establish uniform reporting regulations for occupational therapy services, uniform terminology has evolved to encompass facilitating consistency in terminology and in describing the focus of practice. Nonetheless, the extent to which uniform terminology has actually filtered into practice is questionable. When practitioners were asked to describe the deficits illustrated in a case narrative, the results indicated a low level of agreement between their descriptions and those of the uniform terminology (Borst & Nelson, 1993).

Uniformity in stating the occupational therapy diagnosis provides practitioners with a vocabulary for thinking and communicating. When practitioner A consults with practitioner B about a client who 'is unable to prepare meals due to a memory impairment, as evidenced by her repeated requests for instructions; inability to remember whether she salted the soup; failure to remove the soup when it boiled; and burning the corners of the potholder, secondary to traumatic brain injury,' practitioner B can search through his or her 'schemas' to see if he or she has ever treated a client with this occupational therapy diagnosis. If practitioner B identifies clients with an identical or highly similar occupational therapy diagnosis, practitioner B can inform practitioner A about the intervention given and the outcomes obtained. Until occupational therapy practitioners are able to link specific occupational therapy diagnoses with specific occupational therapy interventions that yield specific outcomes, they will not be able to specify what interventions work for which clients.

The development of occupational therapy diagnostic statements would lead logically to the development of diagnostic labels. Initially, each diagnostic statement would be labelled and the statement itself would contain the defining characteristics of that particular occupational therapy diagnosis. Definition allows us to distinguish one type of disability from another type of disability. For example, to define dressing disability is to list the qualities that make it different from other disabilities.

To classify disabilities, however, is to arrange them in groups using a classification principle that takes into account the ways in which they resemble one another. For example, problems might be classified according to occupational areas. Thus, if the occupational areas delineated in the Framework (AOTA, 2002) were used, all disabilities of concern to occupational therapy would be placed in one of seven classifications: activities of daily living, instrumental activities of daily living, education, work, play, leisure, and social participation. In any taxonomic system, the classification principle should be the same. However, a different principle may be used to create sub-classifications. Thus, aetiology might be used as the principle for creating sub-classifications. Accordingly, problems may be further classified as having a sensory, physical, cognitive, affective or environmental aetiology. The classification principle used to create the sub-category would be factors that negatively influence performance. If such a taxonomy were developed, it would be organized using the descriptive (problem) and explanatory (aetiology) components of the proposed occupational therapy diagnostic statement.

A rudimentary classification system for occupational disabilities illustrated with dressing and bathing is outlined in Table 2.2. The first classification principle, occupational area, resulted in the major division of dressing and bathing disabilities. The second classification principle, aetiology, created five major subdivisions based on sensory, physical, cognitive, affective or contextual aetiology. Further subdivisions were created to address the different types of aetiology within each of the five major aetiological classifications. Thus, when reference was made to occupational therapy diagnosis dressing limitation 2b, all practitioners would know that this meant that the client was unable to dress due to inadequate muscle strength.

In the absence of an occupational therapy diagnostic taxonomy to describe clients' functional deficits, the classification system of the World Health Organization has been proposed to serve this function (Townsend *et al.*, 1990). However, when the reliability of clinical judgements involving clients with physical and psychiatric diagnoses was examined using the *International Classification of Impairments, Disabilities and Handicaps* (ICIDH) (WHO, 1980), it was found to be sufficient for survey research but not for clinical practice (Driessen *et al.*, 1995). The revised ICIDH, the *International Classification of Functioning, Disability and Health* (ICF) (WHO, 2001) may function more adequately as a diagnostic taxonomy because it was developed with a rating system in mind. In the ICF, activity limitations and participation restrictions are encompassed in nine domains: learning and applying knowledge; general tasks and demands; communication; mobility; self-care; domestic life; interpersonal interactions and relationships; major life areas; and community, social and civic life. In terms of a diagnostic system, the ICF is a systems model, with three hierarchically organized sub-systems: impairments (body structure and function), activity limitations and participation restrictions, and environmental barriers or hindrances (physical, social, attitudinal). Sub-system components are rated based on the severity of the problem. Activity and participation is also rated in terms of performance or capacity. Questions such as: 'In your present state of health, how much difficulty do you have dressing yourself without assistance?' tap capacity, whereas those phrased as: 'In your present surroundings, how much of a problem do you actually have in dressing?' tap performance. ICF labels and ratings can be readily accommodated in the proposed occupational therapy diagnostic statement. Environmental factors are rated in a manner similar to the other sub-systems.

Table 2.2   Illustrative taxonomy of occupational diagnoses

Diagnostic label	Defining characteristics
Dressing	
Dressing limitation 1	Unable to dress due to sensory impairment
1a	— visual
1b	— tactile
Dressing limitation 2	Unable to dress due to physical impairment
2a	— range of movement
2b	— muscle strength
Dressing limitation 3	Unable to dress due to cognitive impairment
3a	— apraxia
3b	— short-term memory impairment
Dressing limitation 4	Unable to dress due to affective impairment
4a	— apathy
4b	— self-efficacy
Dressing limitation 5	Unable to dress due to contextual limitations
5a	— lack of social support
5b	— architectural barriers
Bathing	
Bathing limitation 1	Unable to bathe due to sensory impairment
1a	— visual
1b	— tactile
Bathing limitation 2	Unable to bathe due to physical impairment
2a	— range of movement
2b	— muscle strength
Bathing limitation 3	Unable to bathe due to cognitive impairment
3a	— apraxia
3b	— short-term memory impairment
Bathing limitation 4	Unable to bathe due to affective impairment
4a	— apathy
4b	— self-efficacy
Bathing limitation 5	Unable to bathe due to contextual limitations
5a	— lack of social support
5b	— architectural barriers

2.4   Relevance to occupational therapy practice

The approach to occupational diagnosis outlined in this chapter begins with the identification of activity limitations or participation restrictions. Hence, it is consonant with the top-down approach to the occupational therapy process (Trombly, 1993). Impairments, negatively influencing performance, are then identified through task analysis. Subsequently, they are evaluated in detail through additional targeted observations or specific impairment tests, such as goniometry for range of movement and screening tests for depression. Then, attention is directed to potential environmental factors restricting performance. Throughout the process, clients collaborate with practitioners to develop an understanding of problems in relation to the client's situation and to prioritize the relative importance of problems.

The top-down approach differs from the bottom-up approach in putting the initial emphasis on occupation. In the bottom-up approach, the practitioner begins the evaluation of performance by exploring impairments. For example, knowing that a client has rheumatoid arthritis, the evaluation may begin with measures of pinch strength. Having ascertained that the client exerts 1.5 pounds of pinch on the right (dominant) and 5 pounds on the left, the practitioner might infer that the client is unable to prepare meals due to inadequate pinch strength. This is a weak diagnostic statement because it is based on a prediction or inference about performance supported by impairment testing but not activity testing.

In this chapter, the cognitive skills required to make accurate occupational diagnoses were stressed. In clinical practice, however, clinical reasoning skills will be ineffective unless they are accompanied by interpersonal and technical skills. Interpersonal skills involve the ability to relate to clients and their families so that they are willing to collaborate with the practitioner in collecting good data, selecting relevant cues, and prioritizing occupational diagnoses. Furthermore, through their attentiveness to clients and the understanding that they demonstrate of the influence of disability on clients' lives, practitioners must foster clients' willingness to not only tell about their performance problems but also show them. The practitioner who establishes and maintains a positive, trusting and therapeutic relationship is more likely to obtain reliable and valid data and to interpret it accurately than one who operates in a neutral or negative practitioner-client relationship.

The technical skills of the diagnostician involve competence in administering diagnostic procedures and tests. Client data are gathered through the senses (vision, hearing, touch, smell, taste, and kinaesthesia) aided by structured and unstructured interviews, observations, and tests. Experience, in and of itself does not impart technical skill. However, practice coupled with self-assessments of performance and validation of one's problem statements by others (e.g. peers, clients) facilitates improvement. Consequently, reflective practitioners with more experience in using specific diagnostic procedures are more likely to administer and interpret them with ease and accuracy than those less practised and reflective.

2.5 Future research

Given the salience of thinking in the occupational therapy process, the dearth of empirical research on clinical reasoning is startling. This is especially the case for diagnostic reasoning because it marks the interface between evaluation and intervention and integrates thinking and action. The current emphasis on out-comes measurement in health care brings the identified connection between problem formulation and outcomes to the forefront of the research agenda.

Rogers (1983) noted that once problems were formulated, clinical reasoning progressed to decisions regarding interventions and outcomes and that the occupational therapy process was marked by a dynamic assessment process in which testing-intervention-retesting were iterative and pervasive (Rogers *et al.*, 1997). This goal oriented problem determination has been supported by Fleming (1991a) and Hagedorn (1996).

Research on how expected outcomes (intervention goals) influence the for-mulation of occupational diagnoses would yield valuable insights into the rea-soning that guides practice decisions. For example, the extent to which matching the expected outcome to the problem clarifies the problem and/or the outcome might be examined. For instance, in intervening for a feeding disability to increase independence, a practitioner may realize that the proposed intervention (use of adaptive equipment and practice to improve hand to mouth performance) may increase independence in feeding, but may fail to improve the client's nutritional status. Thus, evaluation would incorporate measures of food intake in addition to those of feeding performance to ascertain the effects of independence on intake. Hence, the outcome of occupational therapy intervention would be broadened from the performance of an activity (feeding) to the purpose of the activity (adequate nutritional intake).

Diagnosis-outcome research might also spur investigation of the extent to which identified diagnoses become treated diagnoses because of the ease or fea-sibility of achieving them. The relationship between discarded and retained diagnoses and client priorities could then be scrutinized to appraise the client-centredness of one's practice decisions. Alternatively, the implications of practi-tioners' skill in envisioning a client's outcome occupational profile based on the present occupational profile (diagnosis + assets) might be explored. For the out-come to give direction to the diagnosis, practitioners must have an image of what the client can become as a result of therapy (prognosis). Thus, practitioners' skills in 'envisioning' would have a significant influence on problem formulation. In comparisons of novices and experts, experts would be identified as those who achieve the best outcomes as opposed to those who have the most clinical experience. Lastly, problem-outcome research would cause us to question the utility of a pedagogy that teaches evaluation skills in one course and intervention skills in another.

2.6 Conclusion

Occupational diagnosis is a *part* of the reasoning process that underlies the decisions that practitioners make when planning and implementing interven-tions. Historically, the literature reflects a movement from a standard operating mode of thinking, characterized by tradition, procedures and policies, to a problem identification mode, marked by evaluation and solution finding for identified problems. As occupational therapists assumed more responsibility for their services, and services were provided under physician referral as opposed to prescription, a more scientific mode of thinking was required to analyse and synthesize the myriad of data gathered about clients and to make decisions about their care. In diagnostic reasoning, problems are formulated, that is to say diagnosed, and these formulations are summarized as occupational diagnoses. The diagnostic process in occupational therapy continues to be handicapped by the lack of a standardized nomenclature, formula for constructing diagnostic statements and diagnostic classification system. Consequently, it is difficult for occupational therapists to communicate about 'what therapy works best for which patients' and the growth of occupational science is slowed. Evidence suggests that occupational diagnoses are formulated with the goal of intervention in mind, suggesting that the process of diagnosis and prognosis are integrated. Future research on occupational diagnosis should focus on elucidating this linkage.

References

American Occupational Therapy Association (1979). *Occupational Therapy Product Output Reporting System and Uniform Terminology for Reporting Occupational Therapy Services.* Rockville, Md.: AOTA.

American Occupational Therapy Association (2002). *Occupational Therapy Practice Framework Domain and Process, draft XVIII.* Bethesda, Md. AOTA.

Barris, R. (1987). Clinical reasoning in psychosocial occupational therapy: the evaluation process. *Occupational Therapy Journal of Research, 7,* 147–162.

Borst, M.J. & Nelson, D.L. (1993). Use of uniform terminology by occupational therapists. *American Journal of Occupational Therapy, 47,* 611–18.

Day, D.J. (1973). A systems diagram for teaching treatment planning. *American Journal of Occupational Therapy, 27,* 239–243.

Dickoff, J. & James, P. (1975) Theory development in nursing. In: P.J. Verhonick (Ed.), *Nursing Research* (pp. 45–92). Boston: Little, Brown and Co.

Driessen, M.J., Dekker, J., Lankhorst, G.J. & van der Zee, J. (1995). Inter-rater and intra-rater reliability of the occupational therapy diagnosis. *Occupational Therapy Journal of Research, 15,* 259–274.

Elstein, A.S., Shulman, L.S. & Sprafka, S.A. (1978). *Medical Problem Solving: an Analysis of Clinical Reasoning.* Cambridge, Mass.: Harvard University Press.

Fleming, M.H. (1991a). The therapist with the three-track mind. *American Journal of Occupational Therapy, 45* (11), 1007–1014.

Fleming, M.H. (1991b). Clinical reasoning in medicine compared with clinical reasoning in occupational therapy. *American Journal of Occupational Therapy, 45,* 988–996.

Gillette, N.P. & Mattingly, C. (1987). Clinical reasoning in occupational therapy. *American Journal of Occupational Therapy, 41,* 399–400.

Hagedorn, R. (1996). Clinical decision making in familiar cases: a model of the process and implications for practice. *British Journal of Occupational Therapy, 59,* 217–222.

Holm, M.B. & Rogers, J.C. (1989). The therapist's thinking behind functional assessment,

Part II. In: C.B. Royeen (Ed.), *AOTA self study series: Assessing Function*. Rockville, Md.: American Occupational Therapy Association.

Line, J. (1969). Case method as a scientific form of clinical thinking. *American Journal of Occupational Therapy, 23*, 308–313.

McKay, E.A. & Ryan, S. (1995). Clinical reasoning through story telling: examining a student's case story on a fieldwork placement. *British Journal of Occupational Therapy, 58*, 234–238.

Mahoney, F.I. & Barthel, D.W. (1965). Functional evaluation: the Barthel Index. *Maryland State Medical Journal, 14*, 62–65.

Mattingly, C. (1991). The narrative nature of clinical reasoning. *American Journal of Occupational Therapy, 45*, 998–1005.

Medhurst, A. & Ryan, S. (1996). Clinical reasoning in local authority paediatric occupational therapy: planning a major adaptation for the child with a degenerative condition, Part 1. *British Journal of Occupational Therapy, 59*, 202–206.

Munroe, H. (1996). Clinical reasoning in community occupational therapy. *British Journal of Occupational Therapy, 59*, 196–202.

Neistadt, M.F. (1987). Classroom as clinic: a model for teaching clinical reasoning in occupational therapy education. *American Journal of Occupational Therapy, 41*, 631–637.

Newell, A. & Simon, H. (1972). *Human Problem Solving*. London: Prentice Hall.

Parham, D. (1987). Toward professionalism: the reflective therapist. *American Journal of Occupational Therapy, 41*, 555–561.

Reilly, M. (1960). Research potentiality of occupational therapy. *American Journal of Occupational Therapy, 14*, 206–209.

Roberts, A.E. (1996). Approaches to reasoning in occupational therapy: a critical exploration. *British Journal of Occupational Therapy, 59*, 233–236.

Robertson, L.J. (1996). Clinical reasoning, Part 2: Novice/expert differences. *British Journal of Occupational Therapy, 59*, 212–222.

Rogers, J.C. (1983). Eleanor Clarke Slagle Lectureship: 1983; Clinical reasoning: the ethics, science, and art. *American Journal of Occupational Therapy, 37*, 601–616.

Rogers, J.C. & Holm, M.B. (1989). The therapist's thinking behind functional assessment. In: C.B. Royeen (Ed.), *AOTA self study series: Assessing Function*. Rockville, Md.: American Occupational Therapy Association.

Rogers, J.C. & Holm, M.B. (1991). Occupational therapy diagnostic reasoning: a component of clinical reasoning. *American Journal of Occupational Therapy, 45*, 1045–1053.

Rogers, J.C., Holm, M.B. & Stone, R.G. (1997). Evaluation of daily living tasks: the home care advantage. *American Journal of Occupational Therapy, 51*, 410–422.

Rogers, J.C. & Masagatani, G. (1982). Clinical reasoning of occupational therapists during the initial assessment of physically disabled patients. *Occupational Therapy Journal of Research, 2*, 195–219.

Schell, B.A. & Cervero, R.M. (1993). Clinical reasoning in occupational therapy: an integrative review. *American Journal of Occupational Therapy, 47*, 605–610.

Slater, D.Y. & Cohn, E.S. (1991). Staff development through analysis of practice. *American Journal of Occupational Therapy, 45*, 1038–1044.

Strong, J., Gilbert, J., Cassidy, S. & Bennett, S. (1995). Expert clinicians' and students' views on clinical reasoning in occupational therapy. *British Journal of Occupational Therapy, 58*, 119–124.

Townsend, E., Ryan, B. & Law, M. (1990). Using the World Health Organization's International Classification of Impairments, Disabilities, and Handicaps in occupational therapy. *Canadian Journal of Occupational Therapy, 57*, 16–25.

Trombly, C. (1993). Anticipating the future: assessment of occupational function. *American Journal of Occupational Therapy, 47*, 253–257.

Uniform Data System for Medical Rehabilitation (UDS^{MR}). (1996). *Guide for the uniform data set for medical rehabilitation (including the FIM^{TM} instrument)*. Buffalo, NY: Uniform Data System for Medical Rehabilitation.

World Health Organization. (1980). *International Classification of Impairments, Disabilities and Handicaps*. Geneva: WHO.

World Health Organization (2001). *ICF: International Classification of Functioning, Disability and Health*. Geneva: WHO.

Chapter 3
Spirituality in the Context of Occupation: A Theory to Practice Application

Anita M. Unruh, Joan Versnel and Natasha Kerr

3.1 Introduction

Many health professionals have an interest in spirituality, as evidenced in the numerous publications about spirituality in the nursing, psychology, social work, medicine and physiotherapy literature. As Barnes *et al.* (2000) noted, papers about spirituality and religion have appeared in major medical journals, and in the United States more than 30 medical schools have courses about the relationship between spirituality and medicine. In addition to various professional interests, there are institutes or centres that are concerned with fostering commitment to research and professional development in the area of spirituality. For example, in the United States, the Fetzer Institute (www.fetzer.org) and the Center for the Study of Religion/Spirituality and Health (www.dukespiritualityandhealth.org) exist for the promotion of research and education in the area of spirituality and health.

It is important to recognize that interest in spirituality by occupational scientists and occupational therapists differs from the concerns of individuals in the pastoral profession, or spiritual leaders from various faith perspectives. For occupational therapists and occupational scientists, the focus is on the connection between spirituality and occupation. We want to understand the way in which the spirituality of the individual influences the nature of the occupational life of the people we see in practice.

In this chapter, we will discuss the place of spirituality within occupational therapy and occupational science. We will provide an overview of the literature about spirituality in occupational therapy, the current place of spirituality within occupational therapy theory and practice, as well as its relevance to occupational science theory. This section will be followed with a discussion about the relevance

Portions of this chapter first appeared in Unruh *et al.* (2002) and are included here with the permission of the authors and the publisher.

of spirituality to occupational therapy practice. The chapter will conclude with implications for future research of the current knowledge about spirituality.

3.2   Overview of the literature

3.2.1   Definitions of spirituality

There are many efforts to define spirituality. When we reviewed definitions of spirituality in the health literature (Unruh *et al.*, 2002), we found that definitions could be readily categorized as:

(1)   relationship to God, a spiritual being, a higher power, or a reality greater than the self
(2)   not of the self
(3)   transcendence or connectedness unrelated to a belief in a higher being
(4)   existential, not of the material world
(5)   meaning and purpose in life
(6)   life force of the person or integrating aspect of the person
(7)   summative

Although definitions in the first two categories were common, there was a growing tendency in the literature toward secular definitions (categories three to seven) reflecting ideas about transcendence, connectedness, meaning and purpose, and the life force of the individual. Spirituality may have secular, sacred, theistic or religious dimensions depending on the person. We define the differences between these dimensions in Table 3.1.

The secularization of spirituality may reflect a growing tendency in many societies to reject institutional and doctrinal aspects of spirituality that are associated with organized religion (Hill *et al.*, 1998). There are, however, significant objections to this secular trend. Secular definitions may reduce spirituality to something that is no longer meaningful because the element of sacredness is excluded (Hill *et al.*, 1998). McColl (2000, p. 220) maintained that secular definitions are 'dangerously close to psychological constructs'. One could say that many of the ideas in a secular definition, such as meaning and purpose, can be readily discussed without the added layer of spirituality. It is conceivable that issues about meaning for a person may have little to do with anything that we might associate with spirituality. To illustrate this, one of us (AU) heard an interview with a boxer who described in detail his passion and commitment for boxing, describing it much like a flow experience (Csikszentmihalyi, 1990). Although this occupation was clearly meaningful for him, it is difficult to think of boxing as a spiritual occupation. It can be seen, therefore, that meaning and spirituality are not necessarily the same thing. Meaning may be strongly rooted in spirituality, but meaning can also be about something else that is important to the individual. Similarly, it is illogical to argue that religion is separate from spirituality since religious beliefs often deeply shape experiences about transcendence, con-

Table 3.1 Dimensions of spirituality

Dimension	Definition
Secular	Secular refers to concerns with the affairs of this world, that are not sacred or monastic or ecclesiastical (Sykes, 1982, p. 950). We use the term to separate ideas about spirituality that are not related to sacred or religious ideas.
Sacred	Sacred is traditionally defined as 'devoted or held especially acceptable to a deity, dedicated or reserved or appropriated to some person or purpose' (Sykes, 1982, p. 919). This dimension of spirituality infers that there is something greater than ourselves without explicit reference to a belief in a higher being, god, gods, or God.
Theistic	Refers to a 'belief in the existence of gods, or a god, esp. a God supernaturally revealed to man' (Sykes, 1982, p. 1109).
Religious	Religion refers to a 'particular system of faith and worship' (Sykes, 1982, p. 877). Religions often have an explicit and exclusive theistic framework. However, it is possible for a religion to be multifaceted and inclusive of multiple secular, sacred or theistic dimensions of spirituality (e.g. the Universalist Unitarian church).

nectedness, meaning and purpose, and the life force of people who have a particular faith perspective.

3.2.2 Spiritual questioning

Regardless of whether a secular, sacred or religious definition of spirituality is preferred, spirituality implies an active search for answers to fundamental questions about the origin and purpose of human life. Spiritual questions may include: How was the world created? What is the origin of life? Is there life after death? How do we account for the presence of good and evil in the world? Is there a supreme being or a higher intelligence over all life? Why do bad things happen to good people? What are our obligations to each other and the world around us? The nature of the kind of spiritual questions we ask and the way that we search for answers to these questions is shaped by who we are, our environmental context, our life experiences, and our life stages.

Answers to spiritual questions are constructed in many different ways in response to life experiences and the context in which they occur. A religious approach to spiritual questions is often based on a theistic framework within an organized doctrine that sets out answers or teachings in response to spiritual questions. A sacred approach implies that aspects of a theistic framework are rejected but belief in a higher being or ultimate truth may be retained in some way and may guide the search for answers to other spiritual questions. In contrast, a secular approach to the same spiritual questions involves a rejection of religious, theistic and sacred frameworks with a preference for alternative perspectives such as humanism, existentialism, evolution, and so on. The way in which a person approaches spiritual questions influences the beliefs, practices and experiences (Miller & Thoresen, 1999) that are associated with spirituality for the person.

The usefulness of considering the nature of spiritual questions is the clearer separation of the spirituality construct from psychological constructs which may be related but address other aspects of the person. Second, considering the nature of spiritual questions makes it less reasonable to insist on a particular secular, sacred or religious perspective as the professional stance of occupational therapy; it is a personal matter. As a subjective and personal construct, inevitably spirituality must mean what it means to the individual within her or his experience. Whether the profession, or the individual occupational therapist, has a conceptual preference for a secular, sacred or theistic spiritual framework in response to spiritual questioning is secondary. Third, spirituality is not necessarily central in human life; it may be at the core, it may be at the periphery or it may have no relevance to how an individual understands his or her life.

3.3   Current place of spirituality within occupational science and occupational therapy

3.3.1   Occupational science

Spirituality has had more direct discussion in the occupational therapy literature than within occupational science. There are several reasons why this may be so. In Canada, spirituality was introduced into guidelines for practice in the early 1980s. Over time the inclusion of spirituality in documents concerned with practice led to more discussion within the professional literature about the role of occupational therapists in this area. The inclusion of spirituality in practice documents drew urgent attention from educators (e.g. Kirsh *et al.*, 2001), therapists in practice and students (e.g. Russell *et al.*, 1998).

Much of the related research about spirituality in occupational science has been concerned with the meaning and purpose associated with various occupations. Meaning and purpose in this context are related to secular spiritual perspectives. Other researchers have examined diverse views of spirituality within the context of specific occupations (Frank *et al.*, 1997; Howard & Howard, 1997; Unruh, 1997), or occupations as spiritual activity (Howard & Howard, 1997; Toomey, 1999; Luboshitzky & Gaber, 2001). In a thoughtful paper contrasting ideas about doing, being and becoming, Wilcock (1998) elaborated ideas about reflection and contemplation that are tied to ideas that underlie spirituality.

There is an emerging body of research that examines the way in which engagement in occupation facilitates coping with serious health and life crises. These studies suggest that engagement in meaningful occupations can be extremely powerful as a coping strategy. Engagement in occupation in this way may be partially responsive to renewed spiritual questioning during difficult circumstances. Leisure occupations that are associated with enjoyment and renewal (e.g. Heintzman & Van Andel, 1995; Unruh *et al.*, 2000), particularly those that provide an opportunity for reflection, such as gardening, creating art or making music, may be responsive to spiritual needs. There is some evidence from qualitative research that occupations which reinforce perceptions of being normal and healthy at a time when a person's physical health is severely challenged (e.g. Vrkljan & Miller-Polgar, 2001; Unruh & Elvin, 2004) contribute to reconstructing an occupational self. Relationships between spirituality, occupation and occupational identity or occupational self have only recently been considered (e.g. Unruh *et al.*, 2002), and should be examined in future research.

3.3.2 Occupational therapy

As Law *et al.* (1997) have said, spirituality was part of the first occupational therapy writings about practice. But it was not until the 1990s that spirituality received much focused attention. In this time period, there were more than 30 publications. They have covered some of the following issues:

(1) Discussions about spirituality as a domain of concern for occupational therapy (e.g. Egan & De Laat, 1994; Urbanowski & Vargo, 1994; Townsend, 1997; Collins, 1998; Udell & Chandler, 2000; Vrkljan, 2000).
(2) Examination of the relationship between spirituality and occupational therapy from a particular sacred or theistic perspective (e.g. Kelly & McFarlane, 1991a, b; Low, 1997; Rosenfeld, 2001).
(3) Surveys of occupational therapists' perceptions about their role in the area of spirituality (e.g. Engquist *et al.*, 1997; Rose, 1999; McColl, 2000; Taylor *et al.*, 2000).
(4) Ideas about the way occupational therapy interventions might be spiritually based (e.g. Collins, 1998; Townsend *et al.*, 1999; McColl, 2000).
(5) Debates about definitions of spirituality, and the conceptual relationship of spirituality and models for occupational therapy intervention (e.g. Cunliffe, 1994; McColl, 2000; Whalley Hammell, 2001; Unruh *et al.*, 2002).
(6) Education issues with respect to spirituality (e.g. Kirsh *et al.*, 2001).

One of the challenges for occupational therapy theory is conceptualizing the relationship between spirituality and the practice domains of occupational therapy. Canadian occupational therapists have argued that spirituality is a fundamental aspect of human nature and of human occupation (Law *et al.*, 1997) but there has also been criticism of spirituality as the central, core construct in a model of occupation (Whalley Hammell, 2001; Unruh *et al.*, 2002). Many occupational therapists do believe that spirituality must be recognized as important to occupational performance but occupation should be the central concern of occupational therapists. We have argued elsewhere that occupational therapy is fundamentally about occupation rather than spirituality (Unruh *et al.*, 2002).

3.4   Relevance of spirituality to occupational therapy practice

Many occupational therapists and occupational therapy students indicate on surveys that they are unsure about whether or how to approach spiritual matters with their clients (Blain & Townsend, 1993, Engquist *et al.*, 1997; Russell *et al.*, 1998; Rose, 1999; McColl, 2000; Taylor *et al.*, 2000). Secular dimensions of spirituality are less troubling in practice because they draw our attention to familiar issues such as connectedness, meaning and purpose (Unruh *et al.*, 2002). The religious dimension of spirituality generates more discomfort because of the potential to invade rights to privacy or to violate standards that protect cultural and religious freedom of citizens (e.g. Cunliffe, 1994, 1995), or to be drawn into dialogues about beliefs that may differ considerably from one's own beliefs. The perceived promotion of some spiritual views over others through professional publications also challenges occupational therapists' personal convictions (Groom, 1991; Kelly & McFarlane, 1991a, b, c; Cunliffe, 1994, 1995; Kelly, 1995, 1997). Nevertheless, there is also growing acceptance about the inclusion of spirituality within the domains of concern for occupational therapy and interest in further understanding how spirituality might be integrated into professional practice.

3.4.1   Spirituality as occupational therapy intervention

When occupational therapists talk about attending to spirituality in occupational therapy, they tend to conceptualize spirituality as either part of the *process* of occupational therapy or as an *outcome* of occupational therapy. Sometimes spirituality is part of the process *and* the outcome because it is difficult to consider spirituality as an outcome goal without having discussed spirituality in the process of occupational therapy.

Spirituality in the process of occupational therapy intervention

Because client-centred collaboration is central to occupational therapy intervention, occupational therapists talk with the client about what occupations give life meaning. Such discussion may include talking with the client about spirituality and then listening with sensitivity, with compassion, and without hurry to spiritual needs and concerns. Such listening enables the occupational therapist to truly understand what is important and meaningful to the client with respect to spirituality. This discussion may enable the occupational therapist and client to reflect on and prioritize occupational goals for intervention. Sometimes talking about spirituality is explicit, particularly if the discussion is about sacred or religious views of spirituality. At other times spirituality may be implicit and apparent primarily on reflection about the conversation.

The willingness to engage in spiritual discussion is likely to depend on the therapist's own personal comfort with spirituality as well as the nature of the client's spirituality. It may be difficult to talk about spirituality with the client or to attend to the spiritual concerns of clients through enabling occupation if the occupational therapist has not reflected on his or her own personal spiritual views. The spirituality workbook by Townsend *et al.* (1999) contains a variety of exercises that encourage the reader to think about his or her own spirituality and how it might influence daily life and practice. Talking about spiritual matters with clients is facilitated by one's own personal comfort with such issues.

It is important to recognize that personal spiritual views can have a profound impact on the clinical reasoning process occupational therapists use when they interact with clients. Hooper (1997) found that the world view of the occupational therapist, the single subject of this study, was strongly shaped by the therapist's own spirituality. The therapist's world view had a profound impact on his or her clinical reasoning and the decisions he or she made about problem areas and possible interventions. An occupational therapist should always be conscious of the way in which personal spiritual convictions may influence discussion about spirituality with clients.

Spirituality as the outcome of occupational therapy intervention

The opportunity to talk about what really matters to the client can be extremely therapeutic without any further intervention. At other times, discussion about spirituality may identify important needs according to the client's secular, sacred or religious views of spirituality. It may be possible to address spiritual needs through occupation. In this case, a spiritual goal may be a desired outcome of occupational therapy. It is extremely important to note that as an outcome, we refer to the enablement of spirituality from the perspective of the client and not that of the therapist. Second, the intention of the intervention is on enablement of spirituality through occupation rather than to increase, decrease, modify or change the client's spirituality.

Spirituality might be enabled through spiritually-oriented occupational interventions. Many occupations, especially leisure occupations or occupations associated with joy and restorativeness, have a spiritual component for some people some of the time. Playing music, painting, spending time in nature, journal writing or working in the garden may be responsive to a client's spirituality. Enabling the client's ability to participate in such occupations if they are part of the client's spiritual life may enable the client's spiritual well-being. There are many ways in which spirituality might be enabled through occupation. For example, a client with a serious physical disability may feel that playing or listening to music is essential to his or her spirituality, but there may be very little time available for music. Facilitating this occupation may be an important spiritual goal for the client, and may mean closer examination of the client's challenges in occupational performance. The client may prefer to have more assistance and less independence with some occupations in order to have more available time to attend to spiritual needs through music.

Some clients will find spiritual meaning in occupations that are associated with a sacred or religious view of spirituality. Such occupations may include meditation, prayer, singing sacred songs, religious rituals, reading sacred texts, attending spiritual or religious services, and so on. Again, the occupational therapist can work with the client with respect to occupational routines as well as occupational performance issues to provide an opportunity for the client to participate in such activities. Facilitating expression of spirituality through such occupations is highly dependent on the occupational therapist's own personal spirituality and his or her comfort with the spirituality of the client. A therapist should refer to spiritual leaders when the client is clearly searching for spiritual guidance from a spiritual leader, or if a therapist perceives that another person would be better able to attend to the client's spiritual concerns.

3.4.2   Case stories

In this section, we will discuss two case stories and the way in which spiritual needs may emerge in the process of practice. The stories are based on actual clients but the names are fictional.

Cathy's story

Cathy was a four year-old child. She was emotionally withdrawn and developmentally challenged in her ability to learn and in her social skills. She was seen by one occupational therapist for help with her occupational development. Cathy was also referred to a second occupational therapist in an emotional and behavioural programme due to her delayed social skills and emotional withdrawal. Play was used to help Cathy communicate about her needs. In a very early play session, Cathy turned to a doll's house, family doll figures and a Christmas tree, to tell a story about a family Christmas dinner. Following the storytelling about Christmas, the play shifted to a story about an upstairs mother and a new downstairs mother, and a child who went from one to another. Cathy's play parallelled real events in her life. The Christmas dinner was a last memory of her mother who had recently died. Initially Cathy was not told about her mother's death. The story reflected Cathy's unresolved grief for her mother and her ambivalence towards her stepmother. These issues were very difficult for Cathy to express in words and, as yet, they had been given little attention by her father and stepmother.

The spiritual issue in Cathy's story is about connectedness to a mother who was no longer part of her physical life but still had a place in Cathy's emotional life. In this story the issue of spirituality takes a secular form and occurred as part of the *process* of occupational therapy. Spiritual issues of very young children are easily missed because of the child's greater difficulty in communicating his or her inner world to other people. Children may have such needs in response to the death of a family member or when they themselves are faced with a serious life crisis. The child may not have sufficient language or intellectual understanding to use complex affective language or abstract ideas, and yet still experience loss, grief or fear of the unknown. The child may communicate spiritual needs sometimes through words, at other times through behaviour or play.

The occupational therapist attended to spirituality within the process context in which the child presented it. Cathy and her family were referred to a psychiatric social worker for grief counselling. Play was used in occupational therapy with Cathy and her stepmother to foster emotional attachment and facilitate engagement in family occupations.

There was nothing in this story to suggest a sacred or religious aspect to the child's or the family's view of spirituality. The occupational therapist accepted the child's story from a secular spiritual perspective. One of the prominent themes in secular spirituality definitions is spirituality as transcendence and connectedness with others. It is important to note that Cathy's story illustrates the tension between secular perspectives of spirituality and psychological concepts. It is possible to make sense of Cathy's situation as issues about loss and grief without discussion about spirituality. The difficulty with a secular construction of spirituality is this blurring of spirituality with other psychological constructs (McColl, 2000; Unruh *et al.*, 2002).

Karen's story

Karen was 15 years old. She had difficulty living at home with her mother and stepfather, and ran away. When she became pregnant, Karen went back to her home town hoping to rebuild bridges with her family. Sadly, her mother had died suddenly before Karen returned home. Karen was hurt, angry and very uncertain about what plans she wanted to make for herself and her unborn child.

It was, understandably, difficult to form a relationship with Karen. She distrusted adult female figures and initially rejected most attempts to reach out to her. One of the turning points for Karen was the planning of a small funeral service for her mother at her mother's graveside. The service was planned with Karen and included readings from the Bible, a prayer over the grave and planting flowers. With time, Karen was able to address her feelings about her pregnancy, the occupation of parenting, her needs for support and her plans for her child.

Like Cathy, Karen was grieving for a mother. In this situation, a spiritually based occupation helped Karen to begin to deal with her spiritual and emotional crisis. The funeral illustrates a sacred approach to spirituality. Karen said little about her own spiritual views but she drew comfort from a common religious ritual that was familiar. Enabling some degree of spiritual well-being was essential for Karen; she had critical occupational and life decisions to make. The therapist in this situation responded to Karen's spiritual needs because of her collaborative relationship with Karen. She was comfortable with Karen's need for a service of her own for her mother. Had this not been so, the therapist would have discussed with Karen the possible involvement of another health professional or a spiritual leader.

Case story commentary

Both of these stories involve issues about loss and grief, experiences which often engender a spiritual crisis for people. Attending to spirituality requires sensitivity and respect for the client. Because of the subjectivity and profound need that may be associated with spirituality, a therapist must be particularly attentive to the quality of the collaborative relationship and his or her own comfort level with spirituality and with matters of loss.

3.4.3   Ethical issues

The benefits to clients of giving consideration to spiritual matters have been discussed by many occupational therapists (e.g. Egan & De Laat, 1994; Townsend *et al.*, 1999; McColl, 2000). Benefits are much more likely if the client's spiritual views, whether secular, sacred or religious, are respected rather than ignored or challenged, and if care can be provided in such a way that the client's spiritual needs are not violated. A client-centred approach is key to ensure that the spirituality of the client is understood from the client's rather than the occupational therapist's perspective.

As we have discussed elsewhere (Unruh *et al.*, 2002), attending to the spiritual needs of clients relative to their occupational concerns can be harmful as well as beneficial. The spiritual approaches of clients and occupational therapists can easily conflict, particularly when individuals hold strong spiritual convictions. The possibility for conflict and harm is illustrated in the following comments from two respondents in a survey about spirituality and occupational therapy:

> 'I disagree OTs should discuss spirituality with their clients, unless they are of Christian faith. There are too many "religions" out there and they mess up people's minds. Jesus is the only True God.' (Taylor *et al.*, 2000, p. 425)

> 'If any therapists are encouraging any "spirituality" (i.e. New Age, meditation, Moslem, Jehovah's Witness, Mormon, etc.) other than Christ, they are walking in Satanic Spirituality and the forces of evil are alive and well, being encouraged by them. Anything other than Christian spirituality is of the Devil.' (Taylor *et al.*, 2000, p. 425)

The comments of these two occupational therapists reflect strong conservative Christian views. It would be tempting to assume that such conservative views would be likely only among Christians. Nevertheless, any exclusionary spiritual view may cause conflict among individuals who have differing perspectives. The intention of including spirituality in occupational therapy guidelines or models of practice is not to promote one spiritual view over another, nor to provide an opportunity for proselytizing, or conversion of others to particular spiritual perspectives.

Attention to professional obligations and codes of ethics is particularly important in the area of spirituality. Despite attention to a collaborative relationship, the client is usually in a more vulnerable situation relative to the therapist. The client must be protected from actions that interfere with the right to determine his or her own spirituality. Attempting to proselytize or convert a client to one's own spiritual views is an abuse of the professional relationship.

Clients can also be harmed by interpreting the client's needs or experiences as spiritual if the client does not affirm this conceptualization. This approach may cause confusion, resentment, distrust and outright hostility. The imposition of a spiritual perspective can do more harm than good. Providing well-intended spiritual support that is inconsistent with the client's spiritual preferences can be distressing and even offensive.

There are some circumstances when the spiritual views of a family member or a client may cause harm to self or others, as when the spiritual views of parents or caregivers hinder or challenge the provision of care by a health care team for dependent family members. These issues are more likely to concern medical procedures, but may affect occupational therapists as members of a health care team. Such situations typically require involvement of institutional ethics committees.

In summary, an occupational therapist must respect the client's personal and spiritual preferences and must not use the professional relationship to convert clients to his or her own spiritual views. A client has the right not to talk about spirituality with the therapist, and may not consider spirituality as a meaningful construct in his or her life. In some situations, ethical conflicts due to spiritual issues may require the involvement of an institutional ethics committee. Lastly, it is essential that discussion about spirituality with a client is appropriate to the roles and responsibilities associated with the profession of occupational therapy. The occupational therapist should consult or refer to other individuals if the client has spiritual concerns that are beyond the occupational therapist's role or if the occupational therapist perceives that he or she is in possible conflict with the client's spiritual needs.

3.5   Implications for future research

Although there is a long history of interest in spirituality in the occupational therapy literature, we have very limited information about clients' views about spirituality in relationship to their occupational needs. Much more also needs to be understood about the needs of occupational therapy clients with respect to occupational therapy. More work is needed to understand the relationship between spirituality, occupation and occupational well-being. Much of the existing spiritual literature is concerned with values and beliefs. Less is known about the way in which people's occupations influence their spiritual views or their spiritual well-being. In addition to understanding the impact of serious life crises on spirituality, we need a better understanding of the ways in which spirituality might influence well-being through occupational choices and priorities.

In general, spirituality is explored more often in research concerned with palliative care and chronic illness. Very little is known about the way in which spirituality evolves across the lifespan of an individual. There are only a few papers about spirituality and children (e.g. Fulton & Moore, 1995; Hart &

Schneider, 1997; Barnes *et al.*, 2000). There has been little examination of the way in which gender might influence spiritual well-being, distress or the occupations that might be associated with spirituality (see Foley *et al.*, 1998). There is also considerable opportunity to examine spirituality and occupation within a multicultural context that includes diverse ethnic, racial and socio-economic perspectives. There are many opportunities for occupational therapy researchers to contribute to this growing interdisciplinary field.

3.6   Conclusion

In this chapter, we discussed the emergence of spirituality as a key consideration for occupational science and occupational therapy. Much is yet to be discovered about the link between spirituality and occupation, as well as their mutual influences. We defined spirituality as a search for answers to fundamental questions about the origin, and the purpose, of human life. Spirituality may have secular, sacred, theistic or religious dimensions. We also argued that spirituality must be conceptualized from the perspective of the client because of its subjective nature.

It is important to recognize that attention to spirituality in the context of enabling occupation from the perspective that is relevant to the client will be beneficial, but imposition of spirituality that is insensitive or disrespectful of the client's own views and preferences can be harmful. In this chapter, we presented two examples of considering spirituality as process or outcome in occupational therapy intervention.

Future research needs to further explicate the relationship between occupation and spirituality, the influences of both constructs on health and well-being, as well as the developmental and lifespan considerations that have not been addressed in the literature as yet. Occupation and spirituality are part of the fabric of human experience and there is still much to learn about how they are woven together in diverse cultures and contexts.

References

Barnes, L.L., Plotnikoff, G.A., Fox, K. & Pendleton, S. (2000). Spirituality, religion, and paediatrics: intersecting worlds of healing. *Paediatrics, 104,* 899–908.

Blain, J. & Townsend, E. (1993). Occupational therapy guidelines for client-centred practice: impact study findings. *Canadian Journal of Occupational Therapy, 60,* 271–285.

Collins, M. (1998). Occupational therapy and spirituality: reflecting on quality of experience in therapeutic interventions. *British Journal of Occupational Therapy, 61,* 280–284.

Csikszentmihalyi, M. (1990). *Flow: the Psychology of Optimal Experience.* New York: Harper & Row.

Cunliffe, M.W. (1994). Rights, ethics, and the spirit of occupation. *British Journal of Occupational Therapy, 57,* 481–482.

Cunliffe, M.W. (1995). Letters to the Editor: Rights, ethics and the spirit of occupation. *British Journal of Occupational Therapy, 58*, 128–129.

Egan, M. & De Laat, M.D. (1994). Considering spirituality in occupational therapy practice. *Canadian Journal of Occupational Therapy, 61*, 95–101.

Engquist, D.E., Short-De Graff, M., Gliner, J. & Oltjenbruns, K. (1997). Occupational therapists' beliefs and practices with regard to spirituality and therapy. *American Journal of Occupational Therapy, 51*, 173–180.

Foley, L., Wagner, J. & Waskel, S.A. (1998). Spirituality in the lives of older women. *Journal of Women and Aging, 10* (2), 85–91.

Frank, G., Grenardo, C.S., Propper, S., Noguchi, F., Lipman, C., Maulhardt, B. & Weitze, L. (1997). Jewish spirituality through actions in time: daily occupations of young orthodox Jewish couples in Los Angeles. *American Journal of Occupational Therapy, 51*, 199–206.

Fulton, R.B. & Moore, C.M. (1995). Spiritual care of the school-aged child with a chronic condition. *Journal of Paediatric Nursing, 10*, 224–231.

Groom, M. (1991). Letters to the Editor: Zen in the art of occupational therapy. *British Journal of Occupational Therapy, 54*, 233.

Hart, D. & Schneider, D. (1997). Spiritual care for children with cancer. *Seminars in Oncology Nursing, 13*, 263–270.

Heintzman, P. & Van Andel, G. (1995). Research update: leisure and spirituality. *Parks and Recreations, 30* (3), 22, 24, 27–28, 30.

Hill, P.C., Pargament, K.I., Swyers, J.P., Hill, R.L., McCullough, M.E., Hood, R.W. & Baumeister, R.F. (1998). Definitions of religion and spirituality. In: D.B. Larson, J.P. Swyers & M.E. McCullough (Eds), *Scientific Research on Spirituality and Health: a Consensus Report* (pp. 14–30). Rockville, Md.: National Institute for Health Care Research.

Hooper, B. (1997). The relationship between pretheoretical assumptions and clinical reasoning. *American Journal of Occupational Therapy, 51*, 328–338.

Howard, B.S. & Howard, J.R. (1997). Occupation as spiritual activity. *American Journal of Occupational Therapy, 51*, 181–185.

Kelly, G. (1995). Rights, ethics and the spirit of occupation. *British Journal of Occupational Therapy, 58*, 176.

Kelly, G. (1997). Letter to the Editor. The last 60 years. *British Journal of Occupational Therapy, 60*, 436–439.

Kelly, G. & McFarlane, H. (1991a). Zen and the art of occupational therapy: Part 1. *British Journal of Occupational Therapy, 54*, 95–100.

Kelly, G. & McFarlane, H. (1991b). Zen and the art of occupational therapy: Part 2. *British Journal of Occupational Therapy, 54*, 130–134.

Kelly, G. & McFarlane, H. (1991c). Letters to the Editor: Zen in the art of occupational therapy. *British Journal of Occupational Therapy, 54*, 233–234.

Kirsh, B., Dawson, D., Antolikova, S. & Reynolds, L. (2001). Developing awareness of spirituality in occupational therapy students: are our curricula up to the task? *Occupational Therapy International, 8*, 119–125.

Law, M., Polatajko, H., Baptiste, S. & Townsend, E. (1997). Core concepts of occupational therapy. In: Canadian Association of Occupational Therapists, *Enabling Occupation: an Occupational Therapy Perspective* (pp. 29–56). Ottawa, Ontario: Canadian Association of Occupational Therapists.

Low, J.F. (1997). Religious orientation and pain management. *American Journal of Occupational Therapy, 51,* 215–219.

Luboshitzky, D. & Gaber, L.B. (2001). Holidays and celebrations as a spiritual occupation. *Australian Occupational Therapy Journal, 48,* 66–74.

McColl, M.A. (2000). Muriel Driver Lectureship: spirit, occupation and disability. *Canadian Journal of Occupational Therapy, 67,* 217–228.

Miller, W.R. & Thoresen, C.E. (1999). Spirituality and health. In: W.R. Miller (Ed.), *Integrating Spirituality into Treatment: Resources for Practitioners* (pp. 3–18). Washington, DC: American Psychological Association.

Rose, A. (1999). Spirituality and palliative care: the attitudes of occupational therapists. *British Journal of Occupational Therapy, 62,* 307–312.

Rosenfeld, M.S. (2001). Spirituality, motivation and performance. *Occupational Therapy Now, November/December,* 5–9.

Russell, M., Sinclair, H. & Young, H. (1998). Struggling with spirituality in the Canadian Model of Occupational Performance. *The National, 15,* 3.

Sykes, J.B. (Ed.). (1982). *The Concise Oxford Dictionary of Current English* (7th Edn). New York: Oxford University Press.

Taylor, E., Mitchell, J.E., Kenan, S. & Tacker, R. (2000). Attitudes of occupational therapists toward spirituality in practice. *American Journal of Occupational Therapy, 54,* 421–426.

Toomey, M.A. (1999). Reflections on … the art of observation: reflecting on a spiritual moment. *Canadian Journal of Occupational Therapy, 66,* 197–199.

Townsend, E. (1997). Inclusiveness: a community dimension of spirituality. *Canadian Journal of Occupational Therapy, 64,* 146–155.

Townsend, E.T., De Laat, D., Egan, M., Thibeault, R. & Wright, A.A. (1999). *Spirituality in Enabling Occupation: a Learner-centred Workbook.* Ottawa: CAOT Publications ACE.

Udell, L. & Chandler, C. (2000). The role of the occupational therapist in addressing the spiritual needs of clients. *British Journal of Occupational Therapy, 63,* 489–494.

Unruh, A.M. (1997). Spirituality and occupation: garden musings and the Himalayan Blue Poppy. *Canadian Journal of Occupational Therapy, 64,* 156–160.

Unruh, A.M., Smith, N. & Scammell, C. (2000). The occupation of gardening in life-threatening illness. *Canadian Journal of Occupational Therapy, 67,* 70–77.

Unruh, A.M., Versnel, J. & Kerr, N. (2002). Spirituality unplugged: a review of commonalities and contentions, and a resolution. *Canadian Journal of Occupational Therapy, 69,* 5–19.

Unruh, A.M. & Elvin, N. (2004) In the eye of the dragon: women's experience of breast cancer and the occupation of dragon boat racing. *Canadian Journal of Occupational Therapy, 71,* 138–149.

Urbanowski, R. & Vargo, J. (1994). Spirituality, daily practice, and the occupational performance model. *Canadian Journal of Occupational Therapy, 61,* 88–94.

Vrkljan, B.H. (2000). The role of spirituality in occupational therapy practice. *Occupational Therapy Now, March/April,* 6–9.

Vrkljan, B.H., & Miller-Polgar, J. (2001). Meaning of occupational engagement in life-threatening illness: a qualitative pilot project. *Canadian Journal of Occupational Therapy, 68,* 237–246.

Whalley Hammell, K. (2001). Intrinsicality: reconsidering spirituality, meaning(s) and mandates. *Canadian Journal of Occupational Therapy, 68,*186–194.

Wilcock, A.A. (1998). International perspective internationale – reflections on doing, being and becoming. *Canadian Journal of Occupational Therapy, 65,* 248–256.

Chapter 4
Time Use and Disability

Louise Farnworth

4.1 Introduction

Time use concerns the area of social science that focuses on what we do with our time and why. As all human actions are located in time, including past, present and future, time use is a commonality of the human condition. Time can be represented in many ways, for example, clock time versus a temporal experience (Daly, 2001). Throughout this chapter, time use is restricted to the more concrete understanding related to clock time.

Time use surveys in Western industrialized countries provide substantial data that indicate that employed adults have a relatively equal distribution of work, recreational and rest occupations (Castles, 1993; Statistics Canada, 1995; Australian Bureau of Statistics, 1998; Robinson & Godbey, 1999). Because these surveys provide data about the time use of populations, they allow social scientists to compare people across cultures, age, lifestyle and gender and thus, assess social change. In relationship to occupational therapy, analysing how people allocate their time to activities, places and interactions allows us to understand the impact of disability on their participation in activities (World Health Organization, 2001). Thus, comparison of patterns of time use of people with a disability with that of the population as a whole can suggest where their activity participation is restricted or constrained; the disabling consequences of illness (De Vries, 1997). Time use is also an indicator of quality of life (Harvey, 1993). Nevertheless, studying a person's time use has not been central to occupational therapy practice. I argue that information about people's time use will not only assist occupational therapists in the development of intervention programmes, but also in the development of policy that supports fair and equitable access of all people to a range of occupations that lead to or maintain health and well-being.

In relationship to describing terminology, Pierce (2001) has defined the concepts of occupation and activity to facilitate exploration of theoretical relations between the two concepts, to enhance disciplinary discourse and intervention efficacy, moral surety and political strength of the profession. She describes *an activity* as 'a culturally defined, general class of human actions' (p. 139), which enables us to communicate about generalized categories of occupational experiences in a broad, accessible way. Pierce describes *occupation* as 'a specific individual's personally constructed, non-repeatable experience... [It] is a subjective event in perceived temporal, spatial and socio-cultural conditions that are unique to that one-time occurrence' (p. 139). Hence, in the context of time use, activity is a more appropriate concept to use when referring to time use at the population level as it implies that there is some culturally shared idea about categories of action, such as work, self-care and leisure, whereas occupation describes time use at the individual level.

In this chapter, I will discuss the historical and current understandings of the relationship between health and how one uses time. This will be followed by a review of the literature in occupational therapy, and other social sciences, on the time use of people with a disability, and commentary on these findings. I will then critique time use methodology for occupational therapy research and practice. The chapter will conclude by discussing the future contribution of time use studies to supporting occupational therapy's role as a viable health care profession because of our expertise in human occupation.

4.2   Overview

4.2.1   Time use in occupational therapy

Meyer (1922) first espoused that the temporal dimension was the way humans adapt to disability and was a legitimate concern for occupational therapy. He proposed that, 'the proper use of time in some healthful and gratifying activity' (p. 642), is an important aspect in the treatment of any (neuro) psychiatric patient. According to Meyer time reveals itself as a vacuum, inviting us to fill it with doing. He advocated not only that purposeful use of time had the potential to be both health maintaining and health regenerating, but also that the way in which disabled individuals used and organized their time in daily life was a measure of their adaptiveness. In practice, Slagle (1922), a founder of occupational therapy in the United States, organized people with mental illness into 24-hour schedules of a variety of occupations to entrain daily occupational rhythms or habits. Slagle advocated that a complete programme of occupational therapy should include supervised physical training and recreations (e.g. work, exercise and play), all that was considered to constitute normal living (Shannon, 1977). Similarly, in other countries, formative occupational therapy programmes were based on concepts of a balance between different forms of occupation (Jonsson, 1998; Wilcock, 1999a).

In spite of the idea that an individual's time use could be exploited in occupational therapy practice to enhance health, not only was this not subjected to further investigation in occupational therapy research, but such practices also appeared to decline in clinical use. Kielhofner (1977) revitalized these ideas in a seminal paper on temporal adaptation. In that paper, Kielhofner outlined several propositions supporting the notion that temporal functioning was a useful conceptual base from which human adaptation and dysfunction could be better understood. Kielhofner's (1977) propositions included the following:

- A person lives within a cultural context that sets boundaries for competent action and this notion and valuation of time is accumulated by the individual through the process of socialization.
- Humans have a natural temporal order that includes sleep, self-maintenance, work and play. The health of the individual is related to a perceived balance of these occupations that is not only satisfying to an individual, but also for his or her roles in society. These changing roles serve to organize time across the lifespan.
- It is important that the individual's time responds to his or her internalized goals, values and interests.
- Habits are the structures by which daily behaviour is ordered and without them, a person's life would be a chaotic series of disjointed events.
- Temporal dysfunction is compounded by pathology.

For these reasons, Kielhofner proposed that temporal adaptation was a rich conceptual schema for occupational therapy. Unlike other frames of reference it included all aspects of dysfunction impacting on humans and it was a suitable and unifying framework for all areas of practice. As such, he suggested that a temporal conceptual framework could serve the profession well by facilitating the development of evaluations and interventions.

These propositions were subsequently incorporated into a conceptual model of practice for occupational therapists, *A Model of Human Occupation* (Kielhofner, 1985, 1995, 2002). In particular, the principles of temporal adaptation are embodied in the concept of habituation which is defined by Kielhofner (2002, p. 63) as 'an internalized readiness to exhibit consistent patterns of behaviour guided by our habits and roles and fitted to the characteristics of routine temporal, physical and social environments.' Kielhofner (1995, p. 64) suggested that:

'habits and roles weave the patterns with which we typically transverse our days, weeks and seasons; our homes, neighbourhoods and cities; our families, work organizations and communities. In each of these temporal, physical and social contexts, we perform a wide range of occupations. Habits and roles give regularity, character and order to those occupations.'

4.2.2 Time use, occupational balance and imbalance

Occupational therapists and occupational scientists have considered time use as a way to understand a person's balance of occupations that promotes health and well-being (Christiansen, 1996; Wilcock, 1998; Yerxa, 1998; Farnworth, 2000). Christiansen (1996) reviewed three conceptual frameworks for understanding how balance of engagement in occupations impacted on health. The first of these was the way a person used their time. A healthy occupational balance is represented, in much the same way as has been shown by international time use surveys; that the working, healthy adult engages in approximately equal amounts of productive, leisure and self-care activities. A second way of understanding balance is the concept of chrono-biological balance. Christiansen identified that humans have a biological rhythm across the day, our circadian rhythm, in addition to rhythms across the week. These rhythms impact on and are shaped by, what we do and when, and this can affect our health and well-being. In this way, Christiansen implied that there was a clear link between our physiological rhythms (biology), what we do (occupation) and the regularity with which our daily routines take place (habits and routines). A third way of understanding balance is related to whether or not a person's range of daily activities, or goal related occupations, are complementary or in conflict with each other. This notion of balance related to life goals is reflected in the development of personal project analysis (Christiansen *et al.* 1998a, b).

Wilcock also linked occupational balance to biology. She believed that humans need to use time in a purposeful way; it is an important part of a health maintaining process enabling us to meet inborn biological needs, and to exercise mind and body through activities learned and valued by the culture (Wilcock, 1993, 1998, 1999b). She suggested that occupational imbalance:

'involves a state that occurs because people's engagement in occupation fails to meet their unique physical, social, mental or rest needs. It allows insufficient time for their own occupational interests and growth as well as for the occupations each feels obliged to undertake to meet family, social and community commitments.' (Wilcock, 1998, p. 138).

Proposed consequences of occupational imbalance are an increase in boredom, stress or burnout which can lead to negative health symptoms, such as cardiovascular problems, depression, and so on.

4.2.3 Time use, occupation and health

A number of studies have sought to explore the relationship between balance of occupations and well-being for non-working populations (Law *et al.*, 1998). For example, Marino-Schorn (1986) sought to determine whether the amount of time spent by retirees in work, rest or sleep and leisure was related to well-being. She found that participants who spent most of their time in rest and leisure occupations, with very few productive occupations, had lower morale. Similarly, Bird and Fremont (1991) in a follow-up study of the time use of 620 Americans, using time diaries, interviews and a self-rated health survey, found a decreasing positive effect of passive leisure on health. That is, passive leisure improved health up to a point, after which the more the person engaged in passive leisure the more likely the health consequences were negative. Time spent in active leisure was also associated with better health. As with passive leisure, spending time in active leisure improved only up to a point, after which the returns on active leisure became negative. The researchers also found important sex differences in time use and self-rated health. Men spent twice as much time in paid employment and earned more than 3.5 times as much, whereas women spent 3.5 times as many hours per week in household labour than men. As hypothesized, they found that paid work and wages exerted strong positive effects on self-rated health. However, time spent in housework had a negative effect on health.

Passmore (1998) studied the leisure experiences of nearly 1200 Australian adolescents aged 12–18. She found that some forms of leisure contribute positively to personal growth and development, and to maintenance and enhancement of mental health and well-being, while others may lead to negative mental health outcomes. In identifying three typologies of leisure occupations – achievement, social and time-out leisure – Passmore (1998) suggested that, achievement leisure occupations are those that provide challenge, are demanding and require commitment, such as sports and music performances. Engaging in achievement leisure occupations was found to have influenced participants' self-efficacy beliefs and competencies and to have had a direct relationship with self-esteem. Social leisure occupations are those whose primary purpose is to be with others. This form of leisure occupation also supported the development of competencies, particularly in the areas of relationships and social acceptance which positively, albeit indirectly, influenced self-esteem. The purpose of time-out leisure was relaxation, which included watching television, listening to music or other occupations that tended to be socially isolating, less demanding and frequently passive. Time-out leisure occupations neither supported competence nor self-esteem enhancement, and were found to be negatively related to mental health outcomes for this population.

In summary, the assumption that there is a relationship between time use and health was embedded in occupational therapy at the profession's inception. The assumption continues to be evident in theoretical writings of occupational therapists and occupational scientists. As the selected studies illustrate, passive leisure may negatively impact on health in the absence of a balance with other engaging occupations, indicating that such assumptions are supported. How the relationship between time use and health is incorporated into current occupational therapy practice and research will now be discussed.

4.3 Place within occupational therapy and occupational science

4.3.1 The influence of a clinical problem on the use of time, health and well-being

Clark *et al.* (1991) suggested that one of the potential contributions of occupational science to society would be the scientific study of occupation that transcends everyday knowledge, particularly that which has underpinned occupational therapy practice. Several papers written by scholars in occupational science have stated the need for further research on the relationship between time use and adaptation to the demands of living (Farnworth, 1990; Pettifer, 1993; Christiansen,

1994, 1996; Lo, 1996; Parham, 1996; Primeau, 1996a, b). Although there is a wide body of international literature concerning the time use of able-bodied populations, there has been surprisingly little published that has focused on the time use of people with disabilities. Given its potential unifying framework for all areas of occupational therapy practice, its absence is particularly notable.

In general, studies that have focused on the time use of people with disabilities suggest that disability has a negative impact on time use in terms of frequency of activities, higher unemployment and altered time allocation compared with the general population. This is important because people with disabilities have also been shown to experience less satisfaction with their performance of activities.

Some studies have compared the time use of clinical and well populations. For example, in Moss and Lawton's (1982) study of time budgets of older people, those who were more functionally independent spent more time away from home and in obligatory tasks, such as housework, cooking and shopping, than those receiving formal care. Those who were more impaired had a higher level of inactivity (rest and relaxation). This research left questions unanswered about the perceived quality of the time use of any of the groups or about how that time use impacted on health.

Subsequent studies of severely impaired elders who were still living in the community awaiting nursing home accommodation have been completed (Moss *et al.*, 1993; Lawton *et al.*, 1995). Using proxy time budgets (i.e. completed by a caregiver), these studies found that receiving assistance from the caregiver consumed more of the day than did self-reported obligatory activities. For the severely impaired elderly person the greatest proportion of the day was spent in passive activities of resting and listening to television or radio. The social context, that is, who the person was with, indicated that the person was alone 56% of the day and with the caregiver 29%. While these data indicate a paucity of stimulating occupations for the elderly person, they also indicate the potential opportunities for occupational therapy in facilitating caregivers to enrich the occupational opportunities for more functional purposes.

Using the Activity Configuration Log, Yerxa and Locker (1990) compared the self-perceived quality of time use of 15 community based adults with spinal cord injuries with an age and sex matched control group. The participants with spinal cord injuries had a higher rate of unemployment and more daily free time than did their non-disabled counterparts, spent more time each day watching television, relaxing, talking and partying. The group of people without disabilities spent more time participating in paid employment, in community organizations and commuting to work. Although the sample size was small, the time use of this group of people without disabilities was similar to data gathered in population based time budgets (Robinson, 1977), indicating that the group's time use was representative of a larger population. The group of people with spinal cord injuries also spent less time engaged in self-maintenance occupations than the group of people without disabilities, probably because helpers provided assistance in these areas. An additional finding was that the affective quality of particular occupations was related to the affective quality of the whole day. That is, if the day itself was experienced more positively, so too were the particular occupations of that day. This supports the proposition that there is a carry-over experiential effect between occupations engaged in within a day. Rather than each specific occupation having its own particular positive or negative impact, their affective qualities are interdependent.

Pentland *et al.* (1998) also studied the relationships between time use and health and well-being in men with spinal cord injury, using interviews and time diaries. They found that the extent of the disability did not predict the amount of time in personal care, productivity, leisure or sleep. Additionally, the amount of time spent in these occupations did not predict outcomes of life satisfaction, perceived health or adjustment to disability. Rather, the most strongly predictive outcomes in this sample were financial stress and social support. This study illustrates that time use can be a useful, but not exclusive, indicator of health and well-being. It is, therefore, important to consider these other factors when studying the relationships between the use of time and health and well-being.

Studies of the time use and experience of time use of people with a mental illness, both living in the community and in institutions, consistently indicate lives dominated by solitary and passive leisure occupations (Weeder, 1986; MacGlip, 1991; Suto & Frank, 1994; Davidson *et al.*, 1995; De Vries, 1997). For example, Delespaul's work (Delespaul & De Vries, 1987; Delespaul, 1995) in the Netherlands, suggested that people with mental illness spend significantly more time doing nothing compared to a control group selected from census data. Similarly, Hayes and Halford (1996) compared the time use of 16 men with schizophrenia, 16 employed and 16 long-term unemployed men, using the 1987 Australian Bureau of Statistics data (ABS, 1987). They found that unemployed men and those with schizophrenia participated in more passive leisure (for example watching television) than the employed group, while those with schizophrenia participated in fewer social activities, less active leisure and slept more than the other two groups. Thus, this study suggested the time use impact of experiencing a clinical disorder is similar to, but goes beyond that of being unemployed.

Neville (1980) studied the time use of a group of people with short-term psychiatric illness, and found that identifying problems of time management led to being able to identify other potential health problems. For example, one young man spent his day at home watching television because he was embarrassed to go out as he was overweight. His use of time was symptomatic of his weight problem. Studying the use of time here allowed the investigator to consider the context in which his time use was dominated by passive leisure and thus more readily identify the impact of both his mental illness and other difficulties, such as perceived obesity.

Harvey *et al.* (2002) and Shimitras *et al.* (2003) analaysed time use data from over 200 people with schizophrenia involved in Harvey's (1996) epidemiological study in London, UK. They also found that people spent most of their day sleeping, in personal care occupations, such as eating, and passive leisure occupations, such as watching television. Participants attending day centres engaged in more active leisure, less domestic occupations and less passive leisure than those not attending day care centres. Based on a logistic regression analysis, Harvey and colleagues found those with longer illnesses were significantly less likely to be participating in productive occupations such as paid or unpaid work. Neither sex, social opportunities at home, nor negative symptoms predicted participation in productive occupations. Passive leisure participation was only predicted by social opportunities in the home; those who were living alone were significantly more likely to be participating in passive leisure such as watching television. No significant illness-related or socio-demographic predictors of participation in active leisure or social occupations were found.

Harvey *et al.* (2002) concluded from these findings that efforts to assist people with schizophrenia with impoverished lifestyles might usefully focus on enabling them to participate in naturally occurring occupations that foster their social inclusion with peers in the community. Further, they suggested that people with schizophrenia who are most likely to need assistance to pursue more active lifestyles are those with lengthier illness and those living alone. Thus, people's social opportunities as well as their disability may impact on their successful pursuit of healthier lifestyles.

Nikitin and Farnworth (submitted) studied the use of time, employing a time budget methodology supplemented with occupational histories, of a group of institutionalized male forensic psychiatric patients. In comparison to the time use data of the mainstream adult Australian male population from 1997, the forensic participants in this study spent 20% more time in recreation and leisure occupations, such as smoking, watching television, listening to music and reading. They recorded 5% more time in personal care occupations, such as sleeping and eating, little time in domestic activities and no time in employment related occupations. Of their personal care time, 89% was spent sleeping and 78% of the time in recreation and leisure occupations was spent in passive leisure. In general, participants were dissatisfied with their use of time, describing themselves as 'killing time', 'inactive' and 'bored'. Many perceived that the environment created barriers to engagement in relevant and meaningful occupations. As their time use was similar to that of mentally ill people living in the community, this study raises issues concerning the impact of a mental illness on time use, as opposed to the impact of a restricted environment. That is, similar to other studies, it may be that an impoverished environment in which to engage in meaningful occupations may have a more significant impact on time use than having a mental illness.

The research discussed indicates that studying an individual's use of time can indicate the overall adaptation of that individual to the requirements of daily life. Although the specific issue is different, each study suggests, and importantly, could be used to justify, the need for the specialist knowledge and skills of occupational therapists. Hayes (2000) argued that research should be the basis for clinical interventions in evidence-based occupational therapy practice. She called for the profession to provide research-based evidence for established initiatives in clinical practice, rather than expending limited research resources on developing novel and diverse interventions. Accordingly, our expertise in understanding the relevance of time use as a major indicator of a person's quality of life is one significant contribution occupational therapists can make in the health arena. However, consistent with Hayes' view, we need to research this area more fully, to further develop and rigorously justify our clinical interventions based on time use. To do this, we will require trustworthy methodological procedures, the subject of the following discussion.

4.3.2   Methodological considerations on studying use of time

Time use studies have used a variety of methodologies, depending on the aims of the study, and all have strengths and limitations, indicating that a combination of methodologies is likely to produce more trustworthy findings. This section will briefly outline several methodologies that may be used by occupational therapists and occupational scientists in both research and practice.

Time diaries have been used extensively in studying human use of time. The time diary requires the participant to complete a log or diary of the sequence and duration of activities engaged in, typically for 24 hours. All activities are recorded including the start and the finish time in addition to other information such as where, who with and for whom the activity was done (see Figure 4.1). A time diary places people engaged in their daily activities within their natural temporal context. An inventory is used to categorize time use that emphasizes the duration of occupations as the basis for comparing behaviours among sub-populations. For example, the 1997 Australian Bureau of Statistics Time Use Diary (Australian Bureau of Statistics, 1998) included categories of personal care, employment related activities, childcare activities, education activities, voluntary work and care activities, purchasing goods and services, domestic activities, social and community interaction, and recreation and leisure.

Since the early 1960s, national time diary studies have been conducted in nearly all Eastern and Western European countries. Countries including Japan, the Netherlands, Canada, Korea, Finland, Norway and Australia conduct recurring studies every five to ten years. Comparable data sets of categories, or units of analysis of time, have been developed internationally so that people's use of time from several nations can be compared – see Table 4.1 (Robinson, 1977; Szalai, 1977; Robinson *et al.*, 1988; Castles, 1993; Statistics Canada, 1995). Many countries are contributing data to the Multinational Time Budget Data Archive being developed by Gershuny from the United Kingdom. The first national Time Use Survey in the United Kingdom was completed in 2001 (Sturgis & Lynn, 1998).

Because time diaries provide such rich population data on people's time use, they are, as has been illustrated previously, of use for comparisons between people with activity participation restrictions. Anonymized forms of these data are available for use by social scientists with an interest in analysing the national time use data for their own research purposes and so could be made use of by occupational therapists (Bridge *et al.*, 2002). Additionally, when data sets such as the 1997 Australian Time Use Survey include questions concerning time use and disability status, these data have particular significance for occupational therapy researchers and occupational scientists.

DAY 1: 12 noon – 3 pm					
	1 What was your main activity? (Please record all activities, even if they only lasted a few minutes)	**2 Who did you do this for?** (e.g. self, a staff member, a patient, family)	**3 What else were you doing at the same time?** (e.g. therapy, watching TV, eating)	**4 Where were you?** (e.g. shops, gardens, lounge, riding in a bus etc.)	**5 Who was with you?** (e.g. no-one, patients, therapist, friend)
12.00	Getting lunch	Self	Listening to radio	Dining room	Patients/staff
.05	Eating lunch	Self			
.10					
.15					
.20					
.25	Talking	Self	Smoking	Garden	Nurse/patients
.30					
.35					
.40					
.45					
.50					
.55					
1.00	Sleeping	Self	Nothing	Lounge	Patients
.05					
.10					
.15					
.20					
.25					
.30					
.35	Talking to OT	Self	Smoking	Lounge	OT
.40					
.45	Lying down	Self	Thinking		Patients
.50					
.55					
2.00	Watching TV	Self	Smoking	Lounge	Patients
.05					
.10					
.15					
.20					
.25					
.30					
.35					
.40					
.45					
.50	Watching TV	Self	Reading newspaper	Lounge	No-one
.55					
3.00					

Figure 4.1   Example of time use diary.

Table 4.1 Time budgets collected in different countries. Adapted with permission from Harvey & Pentland (1999). Time use research. In: W. Pentland, A. Harvey, M.P. Lawton & M.A. McColl (Eds), *Time use research in the social sciences* (pp. 3–18). New York: Kluwer Academic/Plenum Publishers.

Country	Sponsor	Comparable years
Australia	Australian Bureau of Statistics	1987, 1992, 1997
Canada	Statistics Canada	1986, 1992, 1998
Netherlands	Social Cultural Planning Bureau	1975, 1980, 1985, 1990, 1995
Japan	Nippon Hoso Kyokai	1960, 1965, 1970, 1975, 1980, 1985, 1990, 1995
Japan	Prime Minister's Office	1976, 1981, 1986, 1991, 1996
Korea	KBS	1983, 1985, 1987, 1990, 1995
Norway	Statistics Norway	1970, 1980, 1990
UK	Office for National Statistics	2001

There are different ways that time diaries can be completed. The primary method is to ask the client or research participant to complete a diary over two consecutive days (see for example McKinnon, 1992; Stanley, 1995; Fricke & Unsworth, 2001). Alternatively, the therapist/researcher can ask the person about their previous day. When severely disabled elders were unable to complete time diaries, Moss *et al.* (1993) asked carers to complete such surveys. However, this method has potential limitations, as do observational methods. For example, Moss *et al.* found that carers were not always present so data collected was limited to certain times of the day.

Clinical instruments designed to gather time use information include the Occupational Questionnaire (Smith *et al.*, 1986) and the National Institute of Health (NIH) Activity Record (Gerber & Furst, 1992). Both employ a diary configuration to understand a person's actual or typical activities engaged in over a period of time, for example a day. In the Occupational Questionnaire, the person reports in half-hour blocks for the time they are awake on what activities they were performing. The person rates each activity category as work, leisure, a daily living task or rest. The person is then asked how much he or she enjoys the activity, how important the activity is, and how well he or she performs the activity. These questions are aimed at assessing volitional aspects of the Model of Human Occupation, but also provide data about habits and balance of activities in daily life. The NIH Activity Record was developed for use with people who have a physical disability and asks additional questions pertaining to pain, fatigue, difficulty of performance and whether one rests during the activity. Hence, in addition to the information provided by the Occupational Questionnaire, the NIH Activity Record provides detailed information about how a disability influences performance of everyday activities. In this way, the activity record could be modified to elucidate other information such as perceived satisfaction, experience of well-being, and so on; issues that are of interest to both clinicians and researchers.

Beeper methodologies such as Experience Sampling Method (ESM) (Farnworth *et al.*, 1996) or Ecological Momentary Assessment (Stone *et al.*, 1999) collect data on a person's time use in addition to the person's experience of engagement in occupation that is placed within a physical and social context. ESM lends itself to smaller scale studies while the time use data gathered is comparable with data collected by time use diaries (Robinson, 1985). Its uses are not restricted, however, to research questions on time use (see Kennedy, 1998; Toth-Fejel *et al.*, 1998). Farnworth (2000) used ESM and interviewing to investigate the time use and subjective experiences of young offenders, and found that 78% of their time was spent engaging in passive leisure and self-care occupations, but the dominant experience was that of boredom, particularly while engaged in these occupations. This understanding of the potentially negative health outcomes of engaging in such occupations could be addressed, a finding that may not be advocated on the basis of time use findings alone. ESM research is difficult to undertake with some participants, for example those who are uncomfortable with using electronic technology (such as a beeper, palm pocket computer or programmable watch) or who have poor literacy skills to read and complete forms. (For further examples of ESM research with clients in mental health see: Voelkl & Brown, 1989; De Vries, 1992; Paterson, 1998; Vlachou, 2000).

Qualitative methodologies such as *interviews* can provide rich time use data. They tend to be time consuming and the accuracy of the findings is potentially limited due to selective remembering, reinterpreting and resequencing events. It is also difficult for people who may be unfamiliar with verbal reflection. *Direct observation* is potentially more accurate than interviews but it is expensive and because of the intrusiveness on the observer, may alter the participant's behaviour (Robinson, 1985). For this reason, Nikitin and Farnworth (submitted) used a combination of data collection methods: time use diaries, participant observation and the Occupational Performance History Interview II (OPHI-II). The OPHI-II was designed to gather essential data on a person's occupational life history (Kielhofner *et al.*, 1998). The semi-structured interview is based on the idea that current occupations are a consequence of life experiences and environmental influences. It includes questions about how a person currently uses their time, and how that may differ from their previous use of time.

These methodologies offer occupational therapists several alternative assessment techniques that can contribute further to research on the relationship between time use and a person's health and well-being. Use of triangulation, or strategies for ensuring that a study's findings are not the artefact of a single source, potentially increases the confidence in the validity and authenticity of the data and their interpretations. In keeping with Carlson & Clark (1991), triangulation is also consistent with the argument supporting the development of innovative research methodologies in occupational science. There is much scope for occupational therapists to develop such combinations of methodologies that will address trustworthiness and genuineness of time use data collections.

4.4   Relevance to occupational therapy practice

Focusing on how a person uses their time immediately orients the occupational therapist to occupation-based practices (Law *et al.*, 2002; Pierce, 2003). Since studying time use focuses on the occupations engaged in by the person, time use addresses intact occupations across the day, or longer period. Understanding a person's time use in this way gives access to understanding the person as an occupational being. For example, a therapist may see a child daily for individual therapy. Knowing that this child spends five hours each day in a variety of individual therapies may alert the therapist to incorporate additional occupations to meet the needs of the child, such as outdoor and social occupations that are appropriate for the developmental age of the child.

Depending on the methodology used, studying time use may be limited in taking into account such issues as the person's interests, the environment in which the activity is performed, its relevance and meaning to the person, and the choice and control the person has in the activity; all issues directly related to health and well-being. However, time use based on clock time is a constant that we can measure. It therefore provides a basis for comparison between those who are able to engage in a healthy range of occupations of their own choosing, as opposed to those who, for whatever reason, have a disability, or experience environmental barriers, and those who do not have such choices. For example, a therapist may find that a person wants to rest in bed all day, every day. In being client centred, the therapist may support this client's occupational choice. However, using time use data based on healthy individuals would suggest a loss of skills through lack of use (Farnworth, 2000), and may lead the therapist to challenge the client about possible healthy occupations in which they could engage. Additionally, the focus on occupations across the day and the week may mean the therapist negotiates involving the client in a balance of additional occupations.

Another advantage of using time use data is that it is a way of communicating our area of expertise. Cusick (2001) cautioned occupational therapists in using profession-specific language if we are to communicate effectively both outside and inside the profession. She suggested that, 'we need to look at the language of the world and see what terms suit us without too much tampering' (p. 107). Naming and framing the occupations of clients of occupational therapy as passive leisure or self-care can be explained readily, through reference to relevant research findings, to health outcomes such as boredom (Farnworth, 1998), or how it deviates from the general population data. These concepts are also readily linked to the ICF (WHO, 2001), a universal language concerning health and functioning (Hasselkus, 2000; McLaughlin Gray, 2001). Time use findings could become a significant marketing strategy for occupational therapy; people relate to having too much or too little time to do what they want, and the implications this may have on their health.

4.5   Future research and issues

The biggest issue in studying time use is the tension between taking an activity in contrast to an occupational focus. That is, can enough information be gained from finding out about a person's time use in contrast to that gained from understanding the personal meaning to the individual in engaging in such occupations, and its relationship to health and well-being? In the study of Gay *et al.* (1999), patients living in a forensic environment found resting to be highly meaningful. For some, living with the sorrow, as well as the daily consequences of having committed a serious crime when mentally ill, was like a nightmare. Sleeping on the other hand, allowed one to dream of other life possibilities. The potential to omit the subjective aspects of time use, intimately connected with the well-being of the person, is problematic in time use studies. For this reason, Lawton (1999) suggested that it is important to enquire about the subjective meaning for the person through other means than time budget methodologies. This would be consistent with much research in occupational therapy that is based on small numbers of participants, allowing for qualitative data collections, such as interviews, to be used as an adjunct to more quantitative time use methodologies. However, one must not ignore the benefits of larger scale epide-miological studies on the time usage of people with disabilities, that can be used to support the development of public health policies such as that advocated by Wilcock (1998).

Whilst methodologies for studying time use may have limitations, under-standing a person's use of time is a measurement of health outcome. Fisher (1999) suggested that instruments such as the RAND 36-item Health Status Survey (Ware & Sherbourne, 1992; Hayes *et al.*, 1993) that are used to measure changes in sociability and general well-being among people experiencing various health problems, are underpinned by an attempt to make a generalized assessment of how people use their time. Several questions on the shorter versions of the SF36 such as the depression, anxiety and sociability scale (DAS) (Coxon *et al.*, cited in Fisher, 1999) assess a person's sociability, including the extent to which people feel they should avoid, or are likely to be avoided by, others. These questions assume that a change in health status may also accompany a change in the pro-portion of time respondents spend alone or with other people. Additionally, many of the activities about which people are asked to comment in the SF36, such as participating in strenuous sports, carrying groceries, bathing and dressing, have long been categories of activities people are specifically asked about in time diaries. Fisher (1999) believed that the SF36 differs from existing time diary research interests only in asking specifically about the ability to perform activities rather than a person's engagement in the activity. Fisher suggested that time diaries allow the possibility of improving the quality of generalized health out-come research in three ways:

- Detecting changes in behaviour associated with both the benefits and side effects of treatments in relation to other activities.

- More precisely measuring sociability, fatigue and behaviour related to the way people use their time.
- Offering more precise cost-benefit analyses of the treatments for agencies which make the decision on the funding of treatments for health.

On this basis, she proposed several advantages in using time diaries as an outcome measure. Diaries facilitate the measurement of progressive change in behaviour prior to, during and after intervention, in terms of whether people with a disability are able to perform the activities necessary for independent living, and to achieve a better balance of personal care, productive work, leisure and sleep. Time diaries can tell us about the aggregate frequency of the performance of activities as well as the sequencing across the day. The time diary also measures exactly how much time people spend with others, what they do when they are alone or with others, and where they do these activities. While one may spend time talking with friends on the telephone, another may go to the local senior citizens group to meet with these people. While the same amount of time may be used in socializing, the physical setting and activity engagement level to achieve this social activity, is quite different. These differences may have different health benefits for the individual. In this way, time usage is compared over time and, as has been done in several studies, the time use of the person with a disability can be compared against population norms collected from national time use studies.

Fisher (1999) also suggests that time diaries can be applied to valuing the effects of health intervention. If, for example, a person with a severe mental illness was receiving therapy from an occupational therapist to re-engage in social and productive activities, such as working voluntarily at the local recycling outlet and becoming a consumer advocate, time diary data could provide quantitative data to support the costs, in contrast to the societal gains, for this person's new activities. Finally, Fisher proposes that, because time diaries are a relatively innocuous form of assessment, and not costly to administer, using diaries to study a person's use of time produces results that are directly meaningful to the lived experience of people who complete them. Given occupational therapists quest for suitable outcome measures that detect changes attributable to occupational therapy, time diaries have many advantages.

4.6   Conclusion

The International Classification of Functioning (WHO, 2001) recognizes that restrictions in participation in activities is a measure of disability. I have suggested that studying a person's time use can provide a rich insight into disability from an occupational perspective. Although occupational therapy, since its inception, has had a core interest in time use as an indicator of health and well-being, and there is much evidence on time use available internationally from population based studies, we are yet to fully recognize the potential of this perspective to validate our practice. In this chapter, I have discussed several studies concerned with the time use of people with a disability and methodological strategies for further understanding a person's use of time, for occupational therapy practice and research. While there are some limitations in focusing specifically on time use at the expense of understanding the person-environment interaction (issues to do with relevance, meaning, challenge, novelty, choice, control), there are also many advantages in more fully researching time use for people with a disability. To be able to do this, we need to know, and to understand, the use of occupation for enhancing health and well-being, and support this with research evidence that we can articulate in our practice arenas.

References

Australian Bureau of Statistics (1987). *Information paper: Time Use Pilot Survey, Sydney, May–June 1987* (Cat. No. 4111.1). Canberra: Australian Bureau of Statistics.

Australian Bureau of Statistics (1998). *1997 Time Use Survey* (Cat. No. 4153.0). Canberra: Australian Bureau of Statistics.

Bird, C. & Fremont, A. (1991). Gender, time use and health. *Journal of Health and Social Behavior, 32,* 114–129.

Bridge, K., Farnworth, L. & Fossey, E. (2002). *Mining Population Surveys: Potential Sources of Activity Participation Knowledge for Practice.* Paper presented at the 13th World Congress of Occupational Therapists, Stockholm, June.

Carlson, M. & Clark, F. (1991). The search for useful methodologies in occupational science. *American Journal of Occupational Therapy, 45* (3), 235–241.

Castles, I. (1993). *How Australians Use their Time* (Cat. No. 4153.0). Canberra: Australian Bureau of Statistics.

Christiansen, C. (1994). Classification and study in occupation: a review and discussion of taxonomies. *Journal of Occupational Science: Australia, 1* (3), 3–21.

Christiansen, C. (1996). Three perspectives on balance in occupation. In: R. Zemke & F. Clark (Eds) *Occupational Science: the Evolving Discipline* (pp. 431–451). Philadelphia: F.A. Davis Company.

Christiansen, C., Backman, C., Little, B. & Nguyen, A. (1998a). Occupations and well-being: a study of personal projects. *American Journal of Occupational Therapy, 52* (1), 91–100.

Christiansen, C., Little, B. & Backman, C. (1998b). Personal projects: a useful approach to the study of occupation. *American Journal of Occupational Therapy, 52* (6), 439–446.

Clark, F., Parham, D., Carlson, M., Frank, G., Jackson, J., Pierce, D., Wolfe, R. & Zemke, R. (1991). Occupational science: academic innovation in the service of occupational therapy's future. *American Journal of Occupational Therapy, 45* (4), 300–310.

Cusick, A. (2001). The 2001 Sylvia Docker Lecture: 02 OT EBP 21C: Australian occupational therapy, evidence-based practice and the twenty-first century. *Australian Occupational Therapy Journal, 48* (3), 102–117.

Daly, K. (2001). Introduction – minding the time: toward a theoretical expansion of time in families. In: K. Daly (Ed.), *Minding the Time in Family Experience: Emerging Perspectives and Issues* (pp. 1–16). Oxford: Elsevier Science Ltd.

Davidson, L., Hoge, M., Merrill, M., Rakfeldt, J. & Griffith, E. (1995). The experience of long-stay inpatients returning to the community. *Psychiatry, 58,* 122–132.

Delespaul, P. (1995). *Assessing Schizophrenia in Daily Life: the Experience Sampling Method.* Maastricht: IPSER.

Delespaul, P. & De Vries, M. (1987). The daily life of ambulatory chronic mental patients. *The Journal of Nervous and Mental Disease, 175* (9), 537–544.

De Vries, M. (Ed.) (1992). *The Experience of Psychopathology: Investigating Mental Disorders in their Natural Setting.* Cambridge: Cambridge University Press.

De Vries, M.W. (1997). Recontextualizing psychiatry: toward ecologically valid mental health research. *Transcultural Psychiatry, 34* (2), 185–218.

Farnworth, L. (1990). *Understanding Work, Self-care and Leisure in Human Occupation.* Paper presented at the 10th International Congress of the World Federation of Occupational Therapists, Melbourne.

Farnworth, L. (1998). Doing, being and boredom. *Journal of Occupational Science, 5* (3), 140–146.

Farnworth, L. (2000). Time use and leisure occupations of young offenders. *American Journal of Occupational Therapy, 54,* 315–325.

Farnworth, L., Mostert, E., Harrison, S. & Worrell, D. (1996). The experience sampling method: its potential use in occupational therapy research. *Occupational Therapy International, 3* (1), 1–17.

Fisher, K. (1999). *Potential Applications of Time Use Data for Measuring Health Outcomes.* Retrieved 20 April 2002, from http://www.iser.essex.ac.uk/activities/iatur/

Fricke, J. & Unsworth, C.A. (2001). Time use and the importance of instrumental activities of daily living. *Australian Occupational Therapy Journal, 48,* 118–131.

Gay, J., Farnworth, L. & Alcorn, K. (1999). *The Use of Time and its Meaning for Forensic Psychiatric Patients.* Paper presented at the International Forensic Mental Health Conference, Melbourne, March.

Gerber, L. & Furst, G. (1992). Validation of the NIH Activity Record: A quantitative measure of life activities. *Arthritis Care and Research, 5,* 81–86.

Harvey, A. (1993). Quality of life and the use of time theory and measurement. *Journal of Occupational Science: Australia, 1,* 27–29.

Harvey, A. & Pentland, W. (1999). Time use research. In: W. Pentland, A. Harvey, M.P. Lawton & M.A. McColl (Eds), *Time Use Research in the Social Sciences* (pp. 3–18). New York: Kluwer Academic/Plenum Publishers.

Harvey, C. (1996). The Camden Schizophrenia Surveys. I: The psychiatric, behavioural and social characteristics of the severely mentally ill in an inner London health district. *British Journal of Psychiatry, 168,* 410–417.

Harvey, C., Shimitras, L. & Fossey, E. (2002). Time use of people with schizophrenia living in the community: participation in activities and rehabilitation implications. *Schizophrenia Research, 53* (3 suppl.), 239.

Hasselkus, B. (2000). From the desk of the editor – reaching consensus. *American Journal of Occupational Therapy, 54* (2), 127–128.

Hayes, R. (2000). Evidence-based occupational therapy needs strategically-targeted quality research now. *Australian Occupational Therapy Journal, 47* (4), 186–190.

Hayes, R. & Halford, K. (1996). Time use of unemployed and employed single male schizophrenia subjects. *Schizophrenia Bulletin, 22* (4), 659–669.

Hayes, R., Sherbourne, C.D. & Mazel, R. (1993). The RAND 36-Item Health Survey 1.0. *Health Economy, 2,* 217–227.

Jonsson, H. (1998). Ernst Westerlund – a Swedish doctor of occupation. *Occupational Therapy International, 5* (2), 155–171.

Kennedy, B.L. (1998). Feeling and doing: health and mind-body-context interactions during daily occupations of women with HIV/AIDS. Unpublished PhD thesis, University of Southern California, Los Angeles.

Kielhofner, G. (1977). Temporal adaptation: a conceptual framework for occupational therapy. *American Journal of Occupational Therapy, 31,* 235–247.

Kielhofner, G. (Ed.) (1985). *A Model of Human Occupation: Theory and Application.* Baltimore: Williams and Wilkins.

Kielhofner, G. (1995). *A Model of Human Occupation: Theory and Application* (2nd edn). Baltimore: Williams & Wilkins.

Kielhofner, G. (2002). *A Model of Human Occupation: Theory and Application* (3rd edn). Baltimore: Lippincott Williams & Wilkins.

Kielhofner, G., Mallinson, T., Crawford, C., Nowak, M., Rigby, M., Henry, A. & Walens, D. (1998). *A User's Manual for the Occupational Performance History Interview.* Chicago: Model of Human Occupation Clearinghouse.

Law, M., Baum, C. & Baptiste, S. (2002). *Occupation-based Practice: Fostering Performance and Participation.* Thorofare, NJ: Slack.

Law, M., Steinwender, S. & Leclair, L. (1998). Occupation, health and well-being. *Canadian Journal of Occupational Therapy, 65* (2), 81–91.

Lawton, M.P. (1999). Methods and concepts for time-budget research on elders. In: W. Pentland, A. Harvey, M.P. Lawton & M. McColl (Eds), *Time Use Research in the Social Sciences.* New York: Kluwer Academic/Plenum Publishers.

Lawton, M.P., Moss, M. & Duhamel, L. (1995). Quality of life among elderly care receivers. *Journal of Applied Gerontology, 14,* 150–171.

Lo, J.L. (1996). The relationship between daily occupational affective experiences and subjective well-being. *Occupational Therapy International, 3* (3), 190–203.

MacGlip, D. (1991). A quality of life study of discharged long-term psychiatric patients. *Journal of Advanced Nursing, 16,* 1206–1215.

McKinnon, A. (1992). Time use for self care, productivity, and leisure among elderly Canadians. *Canadian Journal of Occupational Therapy, 59* (2), 102–110.

McLaughlin Gray, J. (2001). Discussion of the ICIDH-2 in relation to occupational therapy and occupational science. *Scandinavian Journal of Occupational Therapy, 8,* 19–30.

Marino-Schorn, J. (1986). Morale, work and leisure in retirement. *Physical and Occupational Therapy in Geriatrics, 4* (2), 49.

Meyer, A. (1922, reprinted 1977). The philosophy of occupational therapy. *American Journal of Occupational Therapy, 31* (10), 639–642.

Moss, M. & Lawton, M.P. (1982). The time budgets of older people: a window on four lifestyles. *Journal of Gerontology, 37* (1), 115.

Moss, M., Lawton, M.P., Kleban, M. & Duhamel, L. (1993). Time budgets of caregiving of impaired elders before and after institutionalization. *Journal of Gerontology: Social Sciences, 48,* S102–S111.

Neville, A. (1980). Temporal adaptation: application with short-term psychiatric patients. *American Journal of Occupational Therapy, 34* (5), 328–331.

Nikitin, L. & Farnworth, L. (submitted). Time use of institutionalised forensic psychiatry patients. *Australian Occupational Therapy Journal.*

Parham, D. (1996). Perspectives on play. In: R. Zemke & F. Clark (Eds), *Occupational Science: the Evolving Discipline* (pp. 71–80). Philadelphia: F.A. Davis Company.

Passmore, A. (1998). Does leisure have an association with creating cultural patterns of work? *Journal of Occupational Science, 5* (3), 161–165.

Paterson, R. (1998). Time use and subjective experience of people with schizophrenia in long-term care. Unpublished Graduate Diploma in Occupational Therapy Thesis, La Trobe University, Melbourne.

Pentland, W., Harvey, A. & Walker, J. (1998). Time use, time pressure, personal stress, mental health and life satisfaction from a life cycle perspective. *Journal of Occupational Science, 5* (1), 14–25.

Pettifer, S. (1993). Leisure as compensation for unemployment and unfulfilling work. Reality or pipe dream? *Journal of Occupational Science: Australia, 1* (2), 20–26.

Pierce, D. (2001). Untangling occupation and activity. *American Journal of Occupational Therapy, 55* (2), 138–146.

Pierce, D. (2003). *Occupation by Design: Building Therapeutic Power.* Philadelphia: F.A. Davis.

Primeau, L. (1996a). Work and leisure: transcending the dichotomy. *American Journal of Occupational Therapy, 50* (7), 569–577.

Primeau, L. (1996b). Work versus nonwork: the case of household work. In: R. Zemke & F. Clark (Eds), *Occupational Science: the Evolving Discipline* (pp. 57–70). Philadelphia: F.A. Davis Company.

Robinson, J. (1977). *How Americans Use Time: a Social-psychological Analysis of Everyday Behaviour.* New York: Praeger Publishers.

Robinson, J. (1985). The validity and reliability of diaries versus alternative time use measures. In: F. Juster & F. Stafford (Eds), *Time, Goods and Well-being.* Ann Arbor: Survey Research Center, Institute for Social Research, University of Michigan.

Robinson, J., Andreyenkov, V. & Patrushev, V. (1988). *The Rhythm of Everyday Life: How Soviet and American Citizens Use Time.* San Francisco: Westview Press.

Robinson, J. & Godbey, G. (1999). *Time for Life: the Surprising Ways Americans Use their Time* (2nd edn). University Park, Pa: Pennsylvania State University Press.

Shannon, P. (1977). The derailment of occupational therapy. *American Journal of Occupational Therapy, 31* (4), 229–234.

Shimitras, L., Fossey, E. & Harvey, C. (2003). Time use of people living with schizophrenia in a North London catchment area. *British Journal of Occupational Therapy, 66* (2), 46–54.

Slagle, E. (1922). Training aides for mental patients. *Archives of Occupational Therapy, 1,* 11–17.

Smith, N., Kielhofner, G. & Watts, J. (1986). The relationship between volition, activity pattern and life satisfaction in the elderly. *American Journal of Occupational Therapy, 40,* 278–283.

Stanley, M. (1995). An investigation into the relationship between engagement in valued occupations and life satisfaction for elderly South Australians. *Journal of Occupational Science: Australia, 2* (3), 100–114.

Statistics Canada (1995). *The 1992 General Social Survey: Cycle 7. Time use.* Ottawa: Statistics Canada.

Stone, A., Shiffman, S. & De Vries, M. (1999). Ecological momentary assessment. In: D. Kahneman (Ed), *Well-being: the Foundations of Hedonic Psychology* (pp. 26–39). New York: Russel Sage Foundation.

Sturgis, P. & Lynn, P. (1998). *The 1997 UK Pilot of the Eurostat Time Use Survey*. London: Office for National Statistics (Government Statistical Service Methodology Series 1).

Suto, M. & Frank, G. (1994). Future time perspective and daily occupations of persons with chronic schizophrenia in a board and care home. *American Journal of Occupational Therapy*, *48* (1), 7–18.

Szalai, A. (1977). *Cross-national Comparative Survey Research: Theory and Practice*. New York: Pergamon Press.

Toth-Fejel, G.E., Toth-Fejel, G.F. & Hedricks, C.A. (1998). Occupation-centred practice in hand rehabilitation using the experience sampling method. *American Journal of Occupational Therapy*, *52* (5), 381–385.

Vlachou, V. (2000). Time use and occupational engagement of people in long-term psychiatric rehabilitation. Unpublished Master of Occupational Therapy Thesis, La Trobe University, Melbourne.

Voelkl, J. & Brown, B. (1989). Experience sampling method in therapeutic recreation research. *Therapeutic Recreation Journal*, *23* (4), 35–46.

Ware, J.E. & Sherbourne, C.D. (1992). The MOS 36-Item Short Form Health Survey (SF-36): I. *Medical Care*, *30*, 473–481.

Weeder, T. (1986). Comparison of temporal patterns and meaningfulness of daily activities of schizophrenic and normal adults. *Occupational Therapy in Mental Health*, *6* (4), 27–45.

Wilcock, A. (1993). A theory of the human need for occupation. *Journal of Occupational Science: Australia*, *1* (1), 17–24.

Wilcock, A. (1998). *An Occupational Perspective of Health*. Thorofare, NJ: Slack.

Wilcock, A. (1999a). The 1999 Sylvia Docker Lecture: Creating self and shaping the world. *Australian Occupational Therapy Journal*, *46* (3), 77–88.

Wilcock, A. (1999b). Biological and sociocultural perspectives on time use studies. In: W. Pentland, A. Harvey, M.P. Lawton & M.A. McColl (Eds), *Time Use Research in the Social Sciences* (pp. 189–210). New York: Kluwer Academic/Plenum Publishers.

World Health Organization. (2001). *International Classification of Functioning and Disability: ICF*. Geneva: World Health Organization.

Yerxa, E. (1998). Health and the human spirit for occupation. *American Journal of Occupational Therapy*, *52* (6), 412–418.

Yerxa, E. & Locker, S. (1990). Quality of time use by adults with spinal cord injuries. *American Journal of Occupational Therapy*, *44* (4), 318–326.

Chapter 5
Occupation and Flow

Jon Wright

5.1 Introduction

The relationship between our health and what we do is complex. Many people may be able to identify occupations that make them feel good and others that make them feel not so good. Understanding how and why occupations impact on well-being will enable occupational therapists to provide effective services to service users and the general public. One theory that may help to unravel the relationship between occupation and health is flow. In her literature review, Emerson (1998) found that flow was associated with increased levels of happiness, self-esteem, role satisfaction, work productivity and satisfaction with life. There is also evidence that suggests flow could have a role in the treatment of people with disabilities such as schizophrenia, although this is somewhat controversial (Csikszentmihalyi, 1992; Gerhardsson & Jonsson, 1996; Emerson *et al.*, 1998).

Flow is a construct that has been developed in the field of psychology, primarily by Mihalyi Csikszentmihalyi (1975). It is Csikszentmihalyi's fascination for people who perform occupations without necessarily receiving any external reward that has provided much of the impetus for his development of the flow construct. Flow has been defined as a subjective, psychological state that occurs when people become so immersed in an occupation that they forget everything except what they are doing (Csikszentmihalyi & Rathunde, 1992). People who experience flow find it so enjoyable that they will want to repeat the experience 'even at great cost' (Csikszentmihalyi, 1992, p. 4). It is highly unlikely that anyone will be consciously aware of seeking out flow experiences. A person is more likely to be aware of wanting to do something that they have found particularly enjoyable in the past. Performance of this chosen occupation may result in a flow experience, a psychological state that has been considered to be the highest level of well-being (Csikszentmihalyi & Mei-Ha Wong, 1991).

Another way of conceptualizing flow is as an intrinsic reward that people receive for performing certain occupations. Csikszentmihalyi and Rathunde (1992) have argued that flow may have a role in human evolution as people who experience a positive state of consciousness when they use their skills to meet environmental challenges could have a selective advantage over others. People who have a better chance of survival would be those who are motivated to meet the challenges presented throughout life by developing new skills. From this perspective, flow is an essential aspect of human experience.

In order to use flow therapeutically, occupational therapists need to know what flow is, when, how and with whom it can be used, and what it is likely to achieve. This chapter will address these areas of interest and provide some insights into flow research. Within the following section the characteristics of flow will be identified, including its positive and negative qualities. The research that has been conducted by occupational therapists will be explored, followed by the difficulties of measuring flow and establishing the flow process. The section will conclude by examining the relationship between flow and schizophrenia.

5.2   Overview

It has been proposed that the flow experience has a number of characteristics. Jackson and Csikszentmihalyi (1999) state that the most important characteristic is the balance between the challenge of the occupation and the skills of the individual. In order to experience flow a person has to be doing something that is sufficiently challenging to make full use of the skills they possess. People who have experienced flow report a feeling of being at one with the movements they are making, a merging of action and awareness. A person who experiences flow has clear goals that they want to achieve and receives unambiguous feedback as to how they are progressing. The occupation requires concentration and a high level of attention. Flow involves becoming so absorbed in the occupation that a person loses self-consciousness and forgets worries or negative thoughts. When experiencing flow a person perceives a sense of control over what they are doing. The perception of time is transformed, so that what may take hours feels like it has been minutes. It is also possible, however, for some people to experience time passing more slowly. Csikszentmihalyi (1975) originally used the term 'autotelic' to describe flow. He adopted the word 'flow' as it was one that so many of the people he interviewed used to describe their experience. Jackson and Csikszentmihalyi (1999) continue to use the word 'autotelic' to describe the last characteristic of flow, an experience in which a person performs an occupation for no other reason than for the enjoyment it brings. In her review article, Emerson (1998) showed that researchers differed in their opinion about whether all of the flow characteristics need to be present in order for the experience to be labelled as flow, or whether some aspects are more defining than others. The problem this presents is that comparisons between studies are difficult because it is unclear whether the researchers are examining the same phenomenon.

Csikszentmihalyi (1992) has stated that flow helps to integrate the self, because the deep concentration that is necessary to experience flow usually results in a well-ordered consciousness. That is, when in flow a person's thoughts, intentions, feelings and senses are focused on the same goal, and this results in the individual's perception of a harmonious experience within themselves, in their relationship with other people and with the world in general. Csikszentmihalyi (1992) considered flow to be important because it makes the present more enjoyable and, while it lasts, the unpleasant aspects of life are forgotten.

Although flow has primarily been regarded as a positive phenomenon, it has also been considered as having negative consequences. Csikszentmihalyi (1992) believed that flow can be misused, for example in juvenile delinquency, where it was thought that delinquent actions are motivated by the need to have flow experiences which are not available in everyday life. Emerson (1998) found evidence that flow theory has been applied to and has influenced the design of rehabilitation programmes for young offenders. The principle behind the use of flow in this situation is that young people seem to have a natural desire to seek out experiences in which they can use and develop their skills within challenging occupations. In situations of occupational deprivation, young people may resort to illegal means of obtaining flow experiences, for example joy riding in cars, as there may be limited opportunities in their environments for occupations that are socially acceptable. Rehabilitation programmes can be designed to help young offenders find socially acceptable means of channelling their desire for flow experiences.

Csikszentmihalyi (1992, p. 62) also noted that flow activities could have an addictive quality which might lead to a situation in which 'the self becomes captive of a certain kind of order and is then unwilling to cope with the ambiguities of life.' It would appear probable that having flow experiences too frequently could affect a person's occupational balance to the extent that it could have a detrimental effect on their well-being. While this argument may seem persuasive, more research is needed to examine the relationship between flow, occupational balance and health.

Although a number of studies have been conducted by Csikszentmihalyi and his associates, there have been relatively few by occupational therapists (Jacobs, 1994; Farnworth *et al.*, 1996; Gerhardsson & Jonsson, 1996; Persson, 1996; Emerson *et al.*, 1998; Persson *et al.*, 1999; Rebeiro & Polgar, 1999). Emerson (1998) and Rebeiro and Polgar (1999) have provided reviews of flow literature and have suggested how flow may be relevant to occupational therapy and occupational science. Jacobs (1994) focused on whether flow was experienced by occupational therapists, as she believed that flow experiences at work would improve job satisfaction, work productivity and help employers retain staff. Other studies have examined the relationship between flow and service users with particular occupational difficulties. The work of Persson and his colleagues has examined flow with chronic pain patients (Persson, 1996; Persson *et al.*, 1999). Research by Gerhardsson and Jonsson (1996) and Emerson *et al.* (1998) has challenged the assumption that people with schizophrenia will not be able to experience flow. Farnworth *et al.* (1996) examined the strengths and limitations of the experience sampling method (ESM), a method believed useful in measuring flow, with occupational therapy students.

It has been suggested that people can experience flow whilst performing almost any occupation provided that the conditions are conducive to deep concentration (Csikszentmihalyi & Rathunde, 1992). A possible weakness in our current understanding of flow is that although this may be true, it seems unlikely that everyone could achieve a flow state from almost any occupation. A possible explanation of why people are not able to experience flow from performing a whole range of occupations is that flow theory has not taken into account the meaning the occupation has for the individual. It is possible that the client-centred nature of occupational therapy may facilitate flow experiences in service users, although research is needed to examine this area.

Despite there being many potential opportunities in which a person could experience flow, it has been thought to be a relatively rare experience in everyday life (Csikszentmihalyi, 1975; Massimini & Carli, 1988; Csikszentmihalyi & Rathunde, 1992). There is, however, some disagreement on this point. Donner and Csikszentmihalyi (1992) state that executives spend approximately 44% of their time at work in flow. Farnworth *et al.* (1996) found that occupational therapy students in their final year of study were in flow 31% of the time. There may be a variety of reasons for these diverse findings. It may be because executives and students have more opportunities for flow than most people. For example, executives may be involved in making decisions that require them to be totally absorbed in what they are doing and they may spend less time than most people participating in boring or routine tasks. Occupational therapy students may prioritize their occupations differently during their final year of study and concentrate on their studies in preference to other occupations that are less likely to produce flow. Alternatively, these diverse findings may be due to the difficulty researchers have in measuring flow and establishing whether what a person has experienced is actually a flow experience.

The ability to establish whether or not a person is experiencing flow is not only of importance to researchers. Occupational therapists may want to establish what impact a particular occupation is having on a person's well-being. If the occupational therapist aims to encourage a flow experience in the service user, it would be helpful for them to know if the aim has been met. One way they may be able to know if an intervention has been successful is by measuring whether a service user has experienced flow.

The measurement of flow is undoubtedly a complex task. It involves trying to measure a subjective psychological state (Csikszentmihalyi, 1975) that is private to each individual and which could be viewed from a physiological, psychological or behavioural perspective. Unfortunately, none of these ways of measuring flow are designed for use in occupational therapy practice. The measurement of flow has undergone several developmental stages and a number of approaches have been used. These approaches have included interviews (Csikszentmihalyi, 1975), a flow questionnaire (Csikszentmihalyi *et al.*, 1993), diaries (Csikszentmihalyi & Csikszentmihalyi, 1988), the Experience Sampling Method (ESM) (Csikszentmihalyi & Larson, 1987) and the Flow State Scale (FSS) (Jackson & Marsh, 1996).

ESM is thought to be particularly useful in describing, in detail, the patterns of a person's daily experience and so is useful in clinical research (Farnworth *et al.*, 1996). It has not been devised for use in a clinical setting and may be problematic due to the lengthy and intrusive process that involves participants completing a form at least seven times each day for one week (Csikszentmihalyi & Rathunde, 1992). The FSS was specifically designed for use in sport and physical activity settings. Perhaps the most practical methods for occupational therapists establishing whether their intervention is leading to flow would be a combination of observation and interview. The occupational therapist would need to observe whether the person is absorbed in what they are doing and would need to question them about their experience at the end of a particular occupation.

An area of particular interest for occupational therapists is the precise nature of flow, including how it begins and what happens during and after a flow experience. As flow has been found to enhance a person's well-being it would be useful for occupational therapists to know the increased likelihood of a service user experiencing flow. From understanding what happens during a flow experience, occupational therapists could gain a clearer understanding as to whether a flow experience was a realistic therapeutic goal. Certainly there is some doubt as to whether certain negative emotions or psychological states, what Csikszentmihalyi (1992) describes as psychic disorders, can affect whether someone experiences flow. For example, if a person experiences pain, fear, rage, anxiety or jealousy, they would be likely to be preoccupied by these feelings and be prevented from experiencing flow (Csikszentmihalyi, 1992).

However, it may be possible for a person experiencing these emotional states to experience flow after a period of engaging in an occupation as a distraction or diversion. There is some evidence that distraction can be used to elevate mood, for example in depression (Fennell & Teasdale, 1984), but the relationship between distraction and flow in these situations has not been examined. In understanding what happens after a flow episode, occupational therapists might be able to predict the outcome of a flow experience and possibly facilitate flow occupations to meet the specific needs of service users. For example, flow experiences that resulted in feelings of relaxation could help an anxious person discover occupations that can reduce their levels of arousal. Alternatively, flow experiences that lead to feelings of elation could also increase a person's volition.

There has only been one study that focuses on the flow process, that is, entering, maintaining and terminating a state of flow and the impact of such an experience (Massimini *et al.*, 1988). In this study, interviews were conducted with people who reported experiencing flow. There were 636 participants (255 men and 381 women) from northern Italy, the United States and Thailand, from a range of socio-economic backgrounds. The interview questions included, for example: how did the experience start, what kept it going once it had started, and how did it feel? This research provided new insights into flow. For example, the absence of distractions, having the right amount of time to perform the occupation, and being in a relaxed, friendly, social environment, were important in facilitating flow experiences.

Although these findings are interesting and may have implications for occupational therapy, they need to be accepted cautiously for several reasons. First, the research was not published in a peer-reviewed journal. Second, the research methods employed for data collection and analysis were not explained clearly. Third, the results do not always reflect what was actually happening during the different stages of flow. Certain quotations have been categorized in a questionable way and the way in which these categories relate to the flow model is unclear. For example, Massimini *et al.* (1988, p. 68) found that it was the performance of the occupation itself that triggered the flow experience. Two quotations given to illustrate this category are as follows:

'The feeling begins as soon as I start praying.' (participant: nun with visual impairment; occupation: praying)

'It starts when the ceremony begins.' (participant: Navajo Indian; occupation: participating in a traditional ceremony)

While each quotation mentions the occupation they are involved in, the question remains as to what was actually happening at the stage that flow began. Within the challenge-skills model, flow is thought to occur where the challenges and skill of an occupation both exceed what is normally experienced by the individual (Csikszentmihalyi & Rathunde, 1992). The flow model also predicts that in order to remain in flow, the challenge of an occupation must increase to compensate for skill development, or alternatively, a person's skills must improve as the occupation becomes more challenging (Csikszentmihalyi, 1992).

It appears unlikely that these participants were describing a situation of skill-challenge balance for two reasons. First, the participants report flow occurring as soon as they begin an occupation, that is, before a time when they are faced with a challenging element of the occupation and prior to them having to perform a particularly demanding skill. Second, it could be suggested that praying, for the nun, and performing in a traditional ceremony, for the Navajo Indian, are not particularly challenging occupations. They are, in fact, likely to be occupations that are very familiar to the individuals concerned. It is unclear whether these participants, when performing these occupations, had increased the challenge of the occupation to increase the skills that they used. The participants' reports of experiencing flow as soon as they began praying or as soon as the ceremony began would appear to make this unlikely. It seems possible that it may not be enough to assume that it is the performance of the occupation itself that began the flow experience. Another possibility is that on each of the occasions the participants were able to attend totally to what they were doing, and that this was not related to the challenges or skills involved.

Csikszentmihalyi (1992) has raised the importance of attention in the experience of flow, and Tolle (1999) has suggested that attention is vital to well-being. Tolle believed that people engage in dangerous activities such as rock climbing because it forces them into the present or 'now'. In the now people are thought to feel intensely alive, free of time, free of problems and free of thinking. These phenomena appear to have many similarities with the characteristics of flow as discussed previously. Tolle (1999) points out, however, that people may tend to rely on dangerous occupations to reach this psychological state when it is possible through other means. Tolle suggests that people need not change what they are doing, but how they are doing it. Thus, a person should pay more attention to the doing of the occupation, rather than the result they want to achieve through it. Tolle (1999, p. 56) suggested that 'as soon as you honour the present moment, all unhappiness and struggle dissolve, and life begins to flow with joy and ease'. If this is correct, occupational therapists may need to pay greater attention to the process of engaging in occupations rather than the outcome, in order to enable people to achieve higher levels of well-being.

The capacity to attend to the experience of occupational engagement has also been at the heart of the debate as to whether or not individuals with severe mental health problems can experience flow. Csikszentmihalyi (1992) posited that when a person has difficulty attending to what they are doing, they would have difficulty in experiencing flow. Hatfield (1989, p. 1143) has described how people with schizophrenia have attentional deficits in that they become 'captured by a stimulus rather than being able to choose what to attend to'. Csikszentmihalyi (1992) believed that being unable to concentrate and attending indiscriminately to everything results in a person with schizophrenia being not only unable to enjoy anything, but also unable to experience flow.

Studies by Gerhardsson and Jonsson (1996) and Emerson *et al.* (1998) have provided evidence that contradicts Csikszentmihalyi's theoretical position. Gerhardsson and Jonsson (1996) observed and interviewed three inpatients with a diagnosis of schizophrenia and found evidence that all of them had experienced flow whilst performing self-chosen occupations. In their study of nine adults with a diagnosis of schizophrenia Emerson *et al.* (1998) found that the participants did experience enjoyment, a sense of accomplishment, were able to concentrate and lose track of time and their worries, and also gain energy, interest and arousal from participating in enjoyable occupations. Emerson *et al.* (1998) speculated on why there are these differences and believe that much depends on whether a person is acutely or chronically ill, what occupations are available to them, and to what extent researchers focus on the individual's understanding of their experiences. The relationship between flow and severe mental health problems needs further research. If people with schizophrenia can experience flow, it would be helpful to examine to what extent these experiences can help them.

5.3   Place within occupational therapy and occupational science

An occupation has been defined as 'a person's personally constructed, one-time experience within a unique context' (Pierce, 2001, p. 138) and through these occupations people can experience flow. Although flow does not originate from occupational therapy theory, it can be seen to be complementary to current theories, particularly regarding how occupations motivate us and improve our occupational performance. For example, within the Model of Human Occupation (Kielhofner, 2002) flow theory can be seen as related to the concept of volition.

Within Kielhofner's (2002) concept of volition are three subsystems: personal causation, values and interests. Flow experiences would appear to influence a person's personal causation, or a person's perception of their personal capacity and effectiveness. Csikszentmihalyi (1992, p. 66) claimed that following flow, the self that the person is reflecting upon is not the same person that existed before the flow experience, because the individual has been 'enriched by new skills and fresh achievement.' Also Kielhofner (2002) suggested that people value engaging in occupations because of a strong desire to avoid boredom. Flow is an antidote to boredom and could be perceived as a way in which a person's value of not wanting to be bored manifests itself. Furthermore, interests are those occupations that a person finds enjoyable or satisfying (Kielhofner, 2002). Flow experiences are, by definition, enjoyable experiences that people will want to repeat (Csikszentmihalyi, 1992).

Kielhofner (2002) and Massimini *et al.* (1988) have emphasized the importance of the environment on a person's experience in different but complementary ways. Massimini *et al.* (1988), as previously highlighted, found that the environment has a role in enabling flow experiences to occur. Kielhofner (2002) acknowledges the importance a challenging environment can have in encouraging attentiveness and optimal performance and also notes the consequences of environments that evoke disinterest and boredom, or environments that can foster feelings of anxiety or hopelessness. These views are consistent with Csikszentmihalyi's original work (1975).

Within occupational science, flow can be seen to fall within the domain that examines the ways in which occupation serves adaptation, or how occupations can promote health and well-being (Clark *et al.*, 1998). Flow theory does not promote the idea that any one particular occupation or pattern of occupations are good for the health of human beings. For occupational scientists flow can be viewed as a phenomenon that can help us to understand how occupations may help people attain the highest level of well-being (Csikszentmihalyi & Mei-Ha Wong, 1991).

Flow theory supports the opinions of occupational scientists who have taken an evolutionary perspective of occupation. Wilcock (1993) has proposed that occupation is an innate, biological need that people have. She stated that occupations have enabled humans to: 'develop skills, social structures and technology aimed at superiority over predators and the environment,' as well as to 'exercise and develop personal capacities enabling the organism to be maintained and to flourish' (Wilcock, 1993, p. 20). Csikszentmihalyi (1993) agrees and has stated that flow encourages evolution by rewarding people who discover new challenges and develop new skills by providing a deep sense of enjoyment.

5.4   Relevance to occupational therapy practice

Farnworth *et al.* (1996) stated that flow is a phenomenon that has been understood, perhaps unknowingly, by occupational therapists since the profession began. From the beginning therapists have analysed, graded and adapted occupations to ensure that their clients could succeed within the limits of their abilities. However, Carlson and Clark (1990, p. 239) have argued that Csikszentmihalyi has 'not only significantly enhanced our basic knowledge of occupation, but has also provided important insights concerning the therapeutic use of occupations to promote life satisfaction and health'.

Carlson and Clark (1990) believe that our knowledge of flow now enables therapists to select and recommend occupations for their clients that are likely to lead to a flow experience, thereby enhancing the person's sense of well-being. Occupational therapists need to select therapeutic occupations that are purposeful and meaningful to the service user and in which the service user will actively participate (Fisher, 1998). Therapeutic occupations are likely to lead to flow experiences as they encourage the total attention of the individual. The evidence to date suggests that in order for occupational therapists to encourage flow experiences they need to ensure that the occupations chosen provide the service user with clear goals, and immediate and unambiguous feedback. Moreover, the individual needs to perceive the occupation as challenging to the extent that they have to maximize the use of their skills. The environment that occupational therapy takes place in will also need careful consideration. Fisher (1998) suggests that therapeutic occupations need to take place within natural environments as much as possible. These environments are more likely to lead to flow if they have no distractions and if they are relaxed and friendly enough for a person to be able to perform an occupation without any fear.

Fisher (1998) has posited that occupational therapy practice which relies on exercise or contrived occupation (where the purpose or goal of the occupation originated from the therapist and the meaning to the service user is minimal) is not legitimate occupational therapy practice. If occupational therapists are practising in this way, flow is likely to have little relevance. Flow is only relevant to occupational therapy practice that is grounded in therapeutic occupation.

Flow is of relevance to occupational therapy because of the potential benefits of a flow experience. Whether all the benefits of flow are known as yet, is unclear, but our current knowledge demonstrates that flow is related to increased levels of happiness, self-esteem, role satisfaction, work productivity and satisfaction with life (Emerson, 1998). It can also be viewed as a psychological state that can increase levels of motivation and permit development of new skills (Csikszentmihalyi & Rathunde, 1992). In situations where occupational therapists are working with service users to address such issues, creating opportunities to experience flow need to be considered.

5.5   Future research and issues

In order that the full potential of flow can be used for service users and the general public, we still need to know more about this phenomenon. Further exploration could provide valuable information to assist in therapeutic settings. Understanding whether there are differences between challenge-skills and 'now' experiences, could lead us to understand why there are differences in the perception of time within flow. It is possible that different processes will be identified under the umbrella of flow and that these processes could have different effects. Knowing how occupation can affect our well-being has clear implications for occupational therapy.

To date, much of the research has been with normal populations that have not identified any particular disabilities. Although there has been some work with people with disabilities, we are still unsure whether flow can be experienced with particular conditions and in what circumstances (Emerson, 1998). If it is found that people with disabilities can experience flow, we will need to explore the therapeutic potential of flow in greater depth. Furthermore, certain relationships between flow and health have not been fully considered. For example, it is possible that flow experiences have an effect on serotonin levels that lead to an elevation in mood. It is also possible that being in a state of flow alters the immune system. If the immune system is enhanced by occupation this could have implications for the treatment of disorders in which the immune system is affected. We need to know more about the relationship between flow, occupational balance and health, and whether or not experiencing flow too often has negative health implications. The measurement of flow is undoubtedly complex, but is crucial in order to facilitate further research. A measurement instrument that occupational therapists could use easily within their everyday practice to identify whether or not their interventions were promoting flow experiences would also be invaluable.

5.6   Conclusion

In order to use flow therapeutically, occupational therapists must be aware that flow is a subjective, psychological state that occurs when people become totally absorbed in what they are doing. Occupational therapists may be able to use flow's potential when their practice is grounded in occupation. They may use flow by selecting therapeutic occupations that are purposeful and meaningful to the service user and in which the service user will actively participate. Our current understanding is that occupational therapists may be able to facilitate flow experiences with people who are able to immerse themselves in their occupations. Helping service users to experience flow, occupational therapists can facilitate their development of new skills and increase levels of motivation and well-being. It could be argued that flow can not only be used as a tool within occupational therapy, but could also play as important a role as diet and exercise within health promotion for the general public. Understanding the potential of flow experiences and enabling such experiences could benefit not only individuals, but also society as a whole.

References

Carlson, M. & Clark, F. (1990). The search for useful methodologies in occupational science. *American Journal of Occupational Therapy, 45* (3), 235–241.

Clark, F., Wood, W. & Larson, E. (1998). Occupational science: occupational therapy's legacy for the twenty-first century. In: M. Neistadt & E. Crepeau (Eds), *Willard and Spackman's Occupational Therapy* (pp. 13–21). Philadelphia, Pa.: Lippincott.

Csikszentmihalyi, M. (1975). *Beyond Boredom and Anxiety: the Experience of Play in Work and Games*. San Francisco: Jossey-Bass.

Csikszentmihalyi, M. (1992). *Flow: the Psychology of Happiness*. London: Rider.

Csikszentmihalyi, M. (1993). *The Evolving Self*. New York: Harper Collins.

Csikszentmihalyi, M. & Csikszentmihalyi, I. (Eds) (1988). *Optimal Experience: Psychological Studies of Flow in Consciousness*. Cambridge, UK: Cambridge University Press.

Csikszentmihalyi, M. & Larson, R. (1987). Validity and reliability of the experience-sampling method. *The Journal of Nervous and Mental Disease, 175* (9), 526–536.

Csikszentmihalyi, M. & Mei-Ha Wong, M. (1991). The situational and personal correlates of happiness: a cross-national comparison. In: F. Strack, M. Argyle & N. Schwartz (Eds), *Subjective Well-being* (pp. 193–212). Toronto: Pergamon Press.

Csikszentmihalyi, M. & Rathunde, K. (1992). The measurement of flow in everyday life: toward a theory of emergent motivation. *Nebraska Symposium on Motivation, 40*, 57–97.

Csikszentmihalyi, M., Rathunde, K. & Whalen, S. (1993). *Talented Teenagers. The Roots of Success and Failure*. New York: Cambridge University Press.

Donner, E. & Csikszentmihalyi, M. (1992). Transforming stress to flow. *Executive Excellence,* February, 16–17.

Emerson, H. (1998). Flow and occupation: a review of the literature. *Canadian Journal of Occupational Therapy, 65* (1), 37–44.

Emerson, H., Cook, J., Polatajko, H. & Segal, R. (1998). Enjoyment experiences as described by persons with schizophrenia. *Canadian Journal of Occupational Therapy, 65* (4), 183–192.

Farnworth, L., Mostert, E., Harrison, S. & Worrell, D. (1996). The Experience Sampling Method: its potential use in occupational therapy research. *Occupational Therapy International, 3* (1), 1–17.

Fennell, M. & Teasdale, J. (1984). Effects of distraction on decision making and effect in depressed patients. *British Journal of Clinical Psychology, 23*, 65–66.

Fisher, A. (1998). Uniting practice and theory in an occupational framework. *American Journal of Occupational Therapy, 52* (7), 509–521.

Gerhardsson, C. & Jonsson, H. (1996). Experience of therapeutic occupations in schizophrenic subjects: clinical observations organized in terms of the flow theory. *Scandinavian Journal of Occupational Therapy, 3*, 149–155.

Hatfield, A. (1989). Patients' accounts of stress and coping in schizophrenia. *Hospital and Community Psychiatry, 40* (11), 1141–1145.

Jackson, S. & Csikszentmihalyi, M. (1999). *Flow in Sports: the Key to Optimal Experiences and Performances*. Champaign: Human Kinetics.

Jackson, S. & Marsh, H. (1996). Development and validation of a scale to measure optimal experience: The Flow State Scale. *Journal of Sport and Exercise Psychology, 18*, 17–35.

Jacobs, K. (1994). Flow and the occupational therapy practitioner. *American Journal of Occupational Therapy, 48* (11), 989–996.

Kielhofner, G. (Ed.) (2002). *A Model of Human Occupation: Theory and Application* (3rd edn). Baltimore: Lippincott Williams & Wilkins.

Massimini, A. & Carli, M. (1988). Systematic assessment of flow in daily experience. In: M. Csikszentmihalyi & I. Csikszentmihalyi (Eds), *Optimal Experience: Psychological Studies of Flow in Consciousness* (pp. 266–287). Cambridge, UK: Cambridge University Press.

Massimini, A., Csikszentmihalyi, M. & Delle Fave, A. (1988). Flow and biocultural evolution. In: M. Csikszentmihalyi & I. Csikszentmihalyi (Eds), *Optimal Experience: Psychological Studies of Flow in Consciousness* (pp. 60–81). Cambridge, UK: Cambridge University Press.

Persson, D. (1996). Play and flow in an activity group – a case study of creative occupations with chronic pain patients. *Scandinavian Journal of Occupational Therapy, 3*, 33–42.

Persson, D., Eklund, M. & Isacsson, A. (1999). The experience of everyday occupations and its relation to sense of coherence – a methodological study. *Journal of Occupational Science, 6* (1), 13–26.

Pierce, D. (2001). Untangling occupation and activity. *American Journal of Occupational Therapy, 55*, 138–146.

Rebeiro, K. & Polgar, J. (1999). Enabling occupational performance: optimal experiences in therapy. *Canadian Journal of Occupational Therapy, 66* (1), 14–22.

Tolle, E. (1999). *The Power of Now: a Guide to Spiritual Enlightenment*. Novato: New World Library.

Wilcock, A. (1993). A theory of the human need for occupation. *Journal of Occupational Science: Australia, 1* (1), 17–24.

Chapter 6
On Watching Paint Dry: An Exploration of Boredom

Cathy Long

6.1 Introduction

'Like watching paint dry' is a commonly used simile for any experience which is found to be dull, unstimulating or just plain boring. The function of a simile is to illustrate the nature of something by making a comparison to something else, but it can also mask the real impact of the experience. Hence, 'like watching paint dry' may diminish the potentially destructive experience of boredom. Boredom is an under-researched phenomenon within occupational therapy literature and, indeed, there seems to be a paucity of research more broadly. Consequently it seems to be a little understood phenomenon. In spite of this, I will try to show that boredom is of relevance to occupational therapy practice, to our clients and possibly to ourselves.

Hutchinson (1998), writing from a user perspective, described her feeling of abandonment and alienation on admission to a psychiatric ward and refers to the relentless tedium of being an inpatient. She also highlights the consequences of some of our professional concerns:

'As far as boredom is concerned, my evaluations highlighted a problem – trained nurses did not consider it to be in their remit to "entertain" patients, and occupational therapists becoming ever more sophisticated and anxious to lose their "stuffed toy" image, would only do so if it was part of a patient's treatment.' (Hutchinson, 1998, p. 17)

As an occupational therapist working on an acute psychiatric ward in the early 1990s, I can remember that reluctance to engage with clients on the sole basis of their needing something to do. Interestingly, wise nursing colleagues avoided using any terms that alluded to boredom when referring people to occupational therapy, having learnt that these were perceived as unacceptable or inappropriate reasons for referral. It is likely that some of the clients on the ward did experience boredom, but as it was a question that was rarely, if ever asked, it is difficult to be sure. Perhaps, more importantly, the extent to which boredom was a characteristic of these people's lives prior to admission, or whether it continued to be a problem on leaving the hospital, was never explored. This also raises questions about how boredom impacts on a person's health and well-being, whether it affects the process of recovery, and if so in what sort of ways.

There are no easy answers to these questions and it is beyond the remit of this chapter to provide definite answers. Rather, the aim is to explore boredom and to tentatively suggest ways in which this applies to working with people in therapeutic contexts. Therefore, the first part of the chapter provides an overview of boredom-focused research, including definitions and factors influencing its occurrence, whilst the second part discusses how this relates to occupational therapy practice. Because boredom is an under-researched area I have tended to rely heavily on a few key articles and for the same reason suggestions for practice are general and tentative.

6.2 Overview

The aim of this first section is to summarize the complex and often conflicting debate regarding definitions of boredom. This will be followed by a discussion of factors influencing its occurrence in relation to the individual, the task, and the environment. Finally, the possible consequences of boredom and how activity has been used as a remedy to it, will be considered.

6.2.1 Defining boredom

It is likely that we can all identify the experience of being bored in ourselves, yet a widely accepted definition of boredom remains elusive. As a consequence there are many and sometimes conflicting opinions as to how to define the phenomenon. For example, it would be reasonable to think that boredom is simply a lack of interest in a subject, situation or activity. However, according to research literature it appears that the experience of boredom is far more complex and perhaps escapes precise classification.

In simple terms, boredom may be defined as being in a state of too low complexity (Mikulas & Vodanovich, 1993). In other words the activity being undertaken is insufficiently demanding in relation to the individual's physical or cognitive capacity. Furthermore Mikulas and Vodanovich (1993) suggest that the resulting state of boredom is necessarily an uncomfortable one. This may be illustrated by considering behaviour associated with the state of being bored: restlessness, pacing, yawning, sighing, fiddling and fidgeting, gazing out of the window, becoming fascinated by minutiae. When boredom is extreme the individual seems to desire to escape either the source of their boredom, or the state itself, finding any distraction to remove themselves from the situation.

> 'To feel bored is to suffer, in however slight a degree and for however short a duration. That is to say it is a state from which one would like to be set free, from which one seeks relief even, perhaps with desperation.' (Healey, 1984, p. 28)

It is important to make a distinction between boredom and depression as there is some evidence that they can appear very similar to each other in that they both involve an absence of interest in activity or in one's circumstances (Barbalet, 1999). However, Barbalet (1999) makes a distinction by suggesting that depression is often inwardly directed towards the self, whilst boredom tends to be outwardly directed towards the activity or the environment.

For most of us the experience of boredom is transient. However, Gabriel (1988) presents case vignettes of adults who experience chronic boredom, a phenomenon which Fisher (1993) labels as pathological boredom. This can be best illustrated by quoting from one of Gabriel's vignettes. Frances recalls:

'When I am bored I feel nothing. Nothing moves me at all. I feel like I am existing and doing nothing but waiting for time to pass, to go by. I just want to finish whatever I have to do. I have had this feeling for years. I don't feel sad but I am not happy. I just feel a sort of nothingness. Nothing interests me.' (Gabriel, 1988, p. 160)

Significantly all of the people Gabriel interviewed made distinctions between their experiences of boredom and depression. Having experienced both, they were able to identify and articulate differences which although seemingly semantic, may highlight some of the inadequacies of the English language in identifying and communicating our precise feelings and experiences. Fisher (1993) suggests that how people recognize boredom and how they use the word to describe what they are experiencing, are of importance when analysing the phenomenon of boredom. This suggests that in a therapeutic context it is worthwhile exploring the client's 'felt' experience of boredom as it is likely that people use the term idiosyncratically.

6.2.2   Factors influencing boredom

All boredom-focused research makes reference to the individual, the environment or the activity when considering causal factors. This concept is not new to occupational therapists in relation to human occupation. For example the person-environment-occupation model (Law *et al.*, 1999) provides a framework for analysing and conceptualizing occupational performance in relation to the complex interaction between these three domains. The extent to which a person is satisfied with their performance is one of the indicators of the degree of fit between person-environment-occupation. In the context of the current discussion, the issue is how boredom, as a subjective experience, influences a person's performance and/or their perception of it. In the interest of clarity the same domains have been used for this subsection but this is not to suggest that the factors fit neatly into one or other category. All of these aspects interact with each other so there is inevitably much overlap between them.

Individual influences on boredom

One important area of study in relation to the individual has been the development of the Boredom Proneness (BP) Scale. Devised by Farmer and Sundberg (1986), it has been used as a means of measuring the extent to which individuals are susceptible to experiencing boredom. The most recent version, as described by Vodanovich and Kass (1990), uses a Likert scale of 28 items, on a self-report basis. Overall, the items emphasize: the extent to which a person feels connected with their environment; their ability to use adaptive resources to overcome feelings of boredom; and their capacity to recognize and use personal competencies.

Vodanovich and Kass (1990) further analysed the items of the BP scale with the purpose of enabling a deeper understanding of the overall score. They suggest that although two individuals may have the same score, the factors underlying their susceptibility to boredom may be very different. For example, one person's scores may indicate fewer personal strategies for effective time use, whilst someone else's may indicate a predominance of working below their competencies. They suggest that having a greater understanding of these underlying factors may be of particular benefit when deciding upon interventions in a therapeutic capacity. Despite this comment the BP scale has been most extensively used with undergraduate students and appears to have had limited application in therapeutic settings. However, there is some tentative evidence which suggests that some people are more vulnerable to boredom than others, at least amongst undergraduate students (Farmer & Sundberg, 1986).

A further aspect associated with personal influences on boredom is the extent to which we attribute meaning to our actions. Barbalet (1999) suggests meaning is not an intrinsic aspect of objects or actions, but it is the person who gives them meaning, and these meanings provide the purpose and context to our actions. Thus, a bored student may not be able to see any relevance in the lecture material and therefore cannot elicit any personal meaning or purpose from their presence in the classroom. Similar findings were reported by Rudman *et al.* (1996) in their study of the meaning senior citizens attached to their occupations. The informants indicated that doing activity promotes the feeling that time is passing quickly, suggesting that their activities helped to alleviate boredom as, when bored, it is usual that time passes all too slowly.

Perkins and Hill (1985) expand on this idea of meaning by making a link between the significance of the activity and the protagonist's motivations. When these are congruent the activity is perceived and experienced as having meaning and is therefore not considered boring. It would be reasonable to suppose that repetitive tasks are generally experienced as boring, but studies have shown that the meaning of the task is more important than monotony (Fiske & Maddi, 1961 cited by Perkins & Hill, 1985). Monotony as a precursor to boredom has been extensively studied, especially in relation to repetitive work-based tasks. However, Perkins and Hill (1985) suggest that monotony is not sufficient for the experience of boredom, as not everyone who is involved with monotonous work feels bored. They hypothesize that it is the person's perception of the work as monotonous which leads to boredom.

Environmental influences on boredom

Fisher (1993), in her discussion of possible causes of boredom in the work place, focused on the relationship between the experience of a task as boring and the external environment. Through her research she found that work colleagues can provide either direct stimulation (through conversation or sharing of a joke) or indirect stimulation (by their mere presence). Thus, it would seem that the social environment of the work place has a role in helping to alleviate boredom. However, some of Fisher's research respondents indicated that they experienced the exact reverse and felt boredom in relation to their co-workers, because they were perceived to be uninteresting or unfriendly, for example. Furthermore she cites research which suggests that the experience of boredom might be subject to social influence: people are more likely to experience a work task as boring if they are told that the task they have been asked to do is routine and unchallenging.

An in-depth ethnographic study by Charlton and Hertz (1989) graphically illustrates how the environment can influence boredom. Their research examined the work of security specialists of the United States Air Force (USAF), whose sole responsibility was to guard nuclear weapons against outside interference. The researchers doubted whether anyone would argue that this was an extremely important job, carrying a huge responsibility, but interviews with the workers highlighted the extreme levels of boredom associated with the role. Although highly trained USAF personnel, their job involved doing nothing for hours on end except observing an unchanging landscape. They perceived their biggest challenge to be one of coping with the unrelenting boredom in a context of a rigid organizational hierarchy, with strict punishments for misconduct.

Even though this is an extreme example, organizations that reduce the amount of stimulation and variety in the work place by imposing inflexible rules (for example, prohibiting talking, giving exact working procedures or limiting the number of breaks from routine) are more likely to engender boredom amongst workers (Fisher, 1993). Likewise, the greater the external control in performing tasks the greater the likelihood of experiencing boredom in relation to it (Fisher, 1993). In other words many work tasks may be experienced as boring simply due to the amount of external pressure to complete the task in a particular way; this seems to take away from enjoyment of the task itself. Similarly, Duncan-Myers and Huebner (2000) studied the relationship between choice and quality of life amongst residents in long-term care facilities. Their findings support previous studies showing that making choices is one way of increasing internal locus of control. Whiteford (1997), in an investigation of time use with a group of inmates in a maximum security prison, found boredom arose from an environment which severely limited opportunities to engage in occupation. Hence, environments which permit and enable individuals to make choices and to have some autonomy, are more likely to provide stimulation and participation, and are therefore less likely to provoke boredom.

Shaw *et al.* (1996) examined the experiences of boredom, time stress (defined as having too little time and too much to do) and lack of choices in the daily lives of adolescents. They suggest that the world is constructed by and for adults, a world from which adolescents are largely excluded. Shaw *et al.* hypothesized that it is this exclusion which leads to adolescents experiencing boredom. One of the aims of their study was to gain insights into the manner in which the dominant adult culture influences and directs the daily lives of adolescents. In school, boredom was more likely to be experienced when the students felt alienated by adult control or authority, for example being put down or humiliated in the classroom. In these situations they seemed to respond by passive non-participation which then led on to feelings of boredom.

Boredom arising from activity

The term 'activity', as opposed to 'occupation', has been used intentionally, as occupation is closely associated with a personal sense of purpose, engagement, value and meaning (Yerxa, 1994; Golledge, 1998; Law *et al.*, 1999). This distinction is particularly important here, as, by definition, boredom is experienced when these core conditions are absent. Indeed a person may not subjectively experience their daily activities as occupations for these very reasons. For example, people who are depressed commonly lose a sense of meaning or purpose in their actions and may experience a sense of disengagement from their occupations.

This suggests that there is a crucial relationship between the individual and the activity which influences the experience of boredom. A brief mention of Csikszentmihalyi and Csikszentmihalyi's (1995) work on flow may help to explain this relationship more fully. They found, through investigation, that people have an intrinsic drive to seek challenges which are greater than their own personal abilities, in order to utilize and further develop their skills. When personal skill and external challenge were equally matched, the subjective experience of the activity improved greatly and intrinsic pleasure was heightened; a phenomenon known as flow. Rebeiro (2001) emphasized flow as an encouragement to occupational behaviour because activities that produce it are more likely to be continued. Also, because flow involves an absorption in an activity, she suggests that awareness of all of life's usual anxieties, monotonies and concerns are less likely to be an intrusion.

Occupational therapy literature emphasizes the importance of personal interest in relation to activity choice and it is reasonable to assume that some personal interest in an object/situation is vital in order to prevent boredom. For example, Matsutsuyu (1969), when establishing a theoretical foundation for an interest checklist, suggested that interests provoke an emotional response which leads us to make choices, and drives us into effective action. Thus, it is the interest which both initiates and maintains action. However, she also suggested that levels of interest can vary in their intensity, most especially when interests become incorporated into the routine of life, and the initial enthusiasm for a particular interest has waned. This indicates that it is possible to feel bored by subjects or activities of personal interest, even if only temporarily. Hence both sources and levels of interest may change over time. Furthermore, there is some suggestion that boredom has a positive role to play in adaptation, being the prompt to our searching out new experiences, ideas or interests by directing us to actions or activities which are more meaningful to us (Vodanovich & Kass, 1990; Barbalet, 1999).

6.2.3   Consequences of boredom

The majority of research in this area focuses on the work place, but even here empirical evidence is limited as tools for measuring boredom are lacking, and boredom is generally ill defined and poorly understood (Fisher, 1993). As a consequence the short- or long-term effects of boredom on health and well-being are largely unknown. However Fisher (1993) indicates that boredom at work can have serious repercussions, for example an increase in numbers of mistakes or accidents, emotional upsets, stress, increased thrill seeking behaviour or risk taking and increased levels of hostility.

Charlton and Hertz's (1989) study demonstrates this, as their research brought to light the ways in which the USAF guards coped with the unrelenting boredom of their work. These ranged from 'authorized' strategies (i.e. those not banned by regulations) to 'high risk' methods. Reading a study manual provided by the Air Force was an example of an authorized strategy. Listening to radios, reading magazines or watching small screen televisions were all restricted activities and subject to severe penalties. In spite of this, many guards participated in this type of activity and described getting more tangible boredom relief from using such high risk methods. Destructive activity was also in evidence as guards described picking holes in the dashboard or seating of patrol vehicles, seemingly as a direct consequence of the stress associated with their boring job. However, these strategies did not appear to eliminate adverse effects to their health and well-being, as the guards pointed to psychological consequences. Some mentioned depression and many talked of difficulty in maintaining morale.

Rule breaking is often assumed to be a consequence of boredom, most especially amongst juveniles, and remains a firmly held belief despite a lack of evidence to support it (Newburn & Hagell, 1994; Farnworth, 2000). Newburn and Hagell (1994) interviewed persistent young offenders and revealed that although a mixture of chaos, sadness and boredom were common characteristics of their lives, a causal link between these experiences and offending behaviour was not found. However, there is some evidence that society can influence boredom, at least among this age group. For example, students who are most bored perceive themselves as least able to meet societal expectations and are often most marginalized by society (Farnworth, 2000).

6.2.4 Occupation as an antidote to boredom

A further theme of direct relevance to occupational therapy practice is how occupation has been used as a remedy for boredom. However, there is limited documented evidence showing how occupation has been used in this way.

As has been shown, Charlton and Hertz's (1989) study indicates some of the strategies the guards adopted to cope with high levels of boredom. However, the study also revealed seemingly pointless activities instigated by superiors to help make time go faster, described by the guards as 'making work'. For example, the guards were made to run around in circles or measure gaps in the fences being guarded. These activities were non-productive in the traditional sense, but given the importance of the task it could be argued that, from the superiors' perspective, the alleviation of boredom by any means was vital.

One study, which illustrates how users of a psychiatric hospital used occupational therapy as a means of relieving boredom, was carried out by Polemni-Walker *et al.* (1992). They explored the reasons why people admitted to a psychiatric hospital participated in occupational therapy groups by comparing views of users of the programmes with those of the occupational therapists facilitating the groups. They found that the widest discrepancy related to 'participation as a diversion from the tedium of the hospital routine', with users rating this more highly than the therapists. Overall the therapists rated the specific therapeutic gains of the programme more highly, for example the development of coping skills. The researchers suggest that there is nothing wrong with the user's diversionary motive, but question whether people who view this as their *primary* reason for participation are gaining the most from occupational therapy. However, Polemni-Walker *et al.* also expressed concern that the users involved in the study were communicating that they did not have enough to do whilst in hospital and that this could have had a negative impact on their recovery.

Perrin (2001) presented a similar argument, albeit with a different emphasis, by highlighting the importance of creativity to life and health, and expressing her sadness that occupational therapists in continuing care settings have moved away from using creative activities with clients. Where creative activity sits in relation to boredom is less than clear, as they are not associated in the literature, but it is likely that, by its very nature, engagement in creative endeavour excludes boredom.

Mee and Sumsion (2001) embraced this notion more fully in their study of users of different community mental health services. Some of the perceived benefits of engagement in occupation that emerged from their interviews reflect some of the themes discussed in this chapter. For example, users reported that the environment helped them find intrinsic motivation and enabled socialization. Having somewhere purposeful to go and fill time in a meaningful way prevented boredom and helped the participants to find meaning in their lives.

In summary, research indicates that boredom is an uncomfortable state of mind, manifested in physical behaviours. Boredom may impact adversely on psychological well-being, but it may also be a driving force for positive action. Boredom may arise from a mismatch between environmental challenge and skill, specifi-cally where the individual is under-challenged in relation to their skill level, or it may arise from incongruity between the activity and the individual's needs, desires or motivations. Environments which allow individuals to exert personal control, make choices or provide opportunities to utilize skills are, according to the literature, least likely to provoke boredom. However, there are also suggestions that some people may be more vulnerable to boredom or have fewer personal capacities to seek out new avenues for stimulation.

6.3   Implications for occupational therapy

This section draws attention to the relevance of the literature discussed previously to occupational therapy practice by proposing general points that may be applied to any health or social care field. It should be noted that none of the following suggestions are new; they all relate closely to best occupational therapy practice. Indeed, it is likely that client-centred occupational therapy unwittingly addresses issues of boredom by, for example, ensuring therapeutic interventions have both meaning and purpose to the client. However, what is different is the conscious acceptance and acknowledgement of boredom as a potential problem for the clients we work with. A discussion of professional considerations follows, with the proviso that the issues surrounding boredom, with regard to particular client groups, environments or interventions require further research.

6.3.1   Environmental factors

It is evident that some environments yield more feelings of boredom than others and that these feelings, especially if prolonged, could have a detrimental effect on a person's health and well-being. For this reason boredom must be a consideration for anyone who is living in restricted and unstimulating environments, as this is where it is likely to be most manifest. Psychiatric inpatient wards, residential accommodation, prisons or other institutions providing long-term care would be examples of these. However, it should be remembered that non-institutional living environments may also restrict occupational opportunities or choices and not having the means to fill time in a meaningful way may be a problem for some clients. For example, people with impaired physical mobility, who find it difficult to get out and consequently have limited access to resources, may find their opportunities for occupational engagement limited and may therefore experience boredom.

Equally, the social environment of therapy is a possible influence of a client's perception and experience of occupational therapy. There are some situations, outpatient settings for example, where clients have an opportunity to discuss their experiences of occupational therapy on an informal basis. It is possible that clients who are bored by their therapy, who do not fully understand its purpose, may negatively influence the perception of others. This is likely to need managing in some way, ideally by working with those who are expressing negativity in order to ascertain how their needs could best be met. Conversely, as all group therapists know, the social environment of the group can, with careful facilitation, encourage participation, motivation and engagement.

6.3.2   Occupational therapy practice

There are at least two ways of viewing the implications for occupational therapy practice. First, is the question of whether or not occupational therapists should simply provide activity as a means of filling the spaces in people's lives. Second, is whether or not the efforts of the profession would be better placed in enabling people to develop more adaptive time use skills. The latter approach is, perhaps, a more valuable and direct means of developing strategies and personal resources which a person could then apply in their everyday life.

Furthermore, it is generally recognized that occupational therapy is in itself a scarce resource and so services need to be allocated with some care according to prioritized need. For example, those people who have limited personal capacities to use resources available to them should, arguably, have our attention more than people who, with the right resources, in a suitable environment would be more able to use time in a meaningful way. This all suggests establishing some means of finding out about how the client experiences boredom, how extensive the problem is and the possible causative factors. One way would be through careful questioning and discussion at the assessment stage.

However, this whole approach fails to help those people whose health or process of recovery may suffer due to the absence of something to do. Herein lies an acute professional dilemma: the extent to which we should provide opportunities for clients to escape the monotony of, for example, hospital routines. For some this may be a very valuable intervention, but it does need consideration in relation to our specific skills and in relation to each particular environment. This is where hard and fast rules are less than helpful. Participation in a low level parallel group while on an inpatient psychiatric ward, for example, might be the starting point for occupational engagement, for some clients. For others the group may provide a diversion from pressing concerns or anxieties. In these circumstances, the client may not be able to aim for more than that, or gain anything more meaningful from the experience. It is also important to remember that periods of quiet contemplation within the therapy process are equally necessary; boredom is not necessarily all bad.

One final thought on our professional dilemma. It would be interesting to investigate whether other health and social care professionals are as concerned, as occupational therapists appear to be, about being perceived as providing boredom relief. For example, would art therapists, clinical psychologists, physiotherapists or others be concerned if their clients perceived their therapy as nothing more than a break from their usual routines? If not, it would indicate that perhaps Hutchinson's (1998) evaluations were right and our dilemma has more to do with wanting to eschew our stuffed-toy image than client need.

6.4   Future research

The majority of research in this area comes from outside hospital and social care settings, and so there is a pressing need for further investigation in relation to these environments, either with users themselves or through health and social care staff. The lived experience of boredom amongst different client groups is undocumented and a better understanding of the issues for particular people and environments would facilitate the development of effective assessment and intervention strategies.

Boredom, from a developmental perspective, has been under-researched and so little is known about how people develop resources to prevent or cope with boredom, and whether strategies change over time. It seems likely, however, that someone at 16 years of age will experience and deal with boredom in a different way to someone who is 70 years of age. Similarly, gender or cultural differences in the experience of boredom, or of the development of personal resources to deal with it, remain unexplored. Again, a greater understanding of how we develop inner resources and of any differences based on gender or culture would help with the progress of effective intervention strategies.

6.5   Conclusion

The ways in which boredom influences people's lives and their occupational performance is little understood, but it is likely to be experienced by some of our clients in some circumstances and may be more of a problem for some than for others. For this reason it is a possible area of intervention for occupational therapists but not necessarily by simply providing activity to fill the gaps in people's lives. This may be a useful intervention for some clients but could perhaps be most effectively provided by other agencies and personnel. For example activity coordinators on inpatient psychiatric wards are in an excellent position to meet this need. Our skills as occupational therapists are perhaps better placed in the development of a bottom-up approach to boredom relief. In other words the development of intervention strategies that enable clients to cope with boredom if it is an ongoing problem, impacting on their health and well-being. However, more research is required before precise recommendations about the nature and design of such strategies can be made.

References

Barbalet, J.M. (1999). Boredom and social meaning. *British Journal of Sociology, 50* (4), 631–646.

Charlton, J. & Hertz, R. (1989). Guarding against boredom: security specialists in the US Air Force. *Journal of Contemporary Ethnography, 18,* 299–326.

Csikszentmihalyi, M. & Csikszentmihalyi, I. (1995). *Optimal Experience: Psychological Studies of Flow in Consciousness.* New York: Cambridge University Press.

Duncan-Myers, A. & Huebner, R. (2000). Relationship between choice and quality in life among residents in long-term care facilities. *American Journal of Occupational Therapy, 54* (5), 504–508.

Farmer, R. & Sundberg, N. (1986). Boredom proneness – the development and correlates of a new scale. *Journal of Personality Assessment, 50* (1), 4–17.

Farnworth, L. (2000). Time use and leisure occupations of young offenders. *American Journal of Occupational Therapy, 54* (3), 315–325.

Fisher, C. (1993). Boredom at work: a neglected concept. *Human Relations, 46* (3), 395–417.

Gabriel, M.A. (1988). Boredom: exploration of a developmental perspective. *Clinical Social Work Journal, 16*, 156–64.

Golledge, J. (1998). Distinguishing between occupation, purposeful activity and activity, Part 1: Review and explanation. *British Journal of Occupational Therapy, 61* (3), 100–105.

Healey, S.D. (1984). *Boredom, Self and Culture*. New Jersey: Associated University Presses.

Hutchinson, M. (1998). Still singing the same old blues. *Health Matters, 34*, 16–17.

Law, M., Cooper, B., Strong, S., Stewart, D., Rigby, P. & Letts, L. (1999). The Person-Environment-Occupation Model: a transactive approach to occupational performance. *Canadian Journal of Occupational Therapy, 63* (1), 9–23.

Matsutsuyu, J.S. (1969). The interest checklist. *American Journal of Occupational Therapy, 23* (4), 323–329.

Mee, J. & Sumsion, T. (2001). Mental health clients confirm the motivating power of occupation. *British Journal of Occupational Therapy, 64* (3), 121–128.

Mikulas, W.L. & Vodanovich, S.J. (1993). The essence of boredom. *Psychological Record, 43* (1), 3–12.

Newburn, T. & Hagell, A. (1994). Arrested development. *Community Care*, 2–8 June, 24–25.

Perkins, R.E. & Hill, A.B. (1985). Cognitive and affective aspects of boredom. *British Journal of Psychology, 76*, 221–234.

Perrin, T. (2001). Don't despise the fluffy bunny: a reflection on practice. *British Journal of Occupational Therapy, 64* (3), 129–134.

Polemni-Walker, I., Wilson, K. & Jewers, R. (1992). Reasons for participating in occupational therapy groups: perceptions of adult psychiatric patients and occupational therapists. *Canadian Journal of Occupational Therapy, 54* (5), 240–247.

Rebeiro, K.L. (2001). Enabling occupation: the importance of an affirming environment. *Canadian Journal of Occupational Therapy, 68* (2), 80–89.

Rudman, D.L., Cook, J.V. & Polatajko, H. (1996). Understanding the potential of occupation: a qualitative exploration of seniors' perspectives on activity. *American Journal of Occupational Therapy, 51* (8), 640–649.

Shaw, S.M., Caldwell, L. & Kleiber, D. (1996). Boredom, stress and social control in the daily activities of adolescents. *Journal of Leisure Research, 28* (4), 274–292.

Vodanovich, S. & Kass, S. (1990). A factor analytic study of the boredom proneness scale. *Journal of Personality Assessment, 55* (1 & 2), 115–123.

Whiteford, G. (1997). Occupational deprivation and incarceration. *Journal of Occupational Science: Australia, 4* (3), 126–130.

Yerxa, E.J. (1994). Dreams, dilemmas and decisions for occupational therapy practice in a new millennium: an American perspective. *American Journal of Occupational Therapy, 48* (7), 586–589.

Chapter 7
Creativity and Occupation

Gaynor Sadlo

'Every moment of your life is infinitely creative' – Shakti Gawain

7.1 Introduction

If some occupational therapists sense a need to bring occupation back into the profession, then perhaps creativity also needs to assume a more central focus, because the two concepts are intimately connected. It appears that the creative treatment methods, such as arts and crafts, which were once popular, are used less often in modern practice. Occupational therapists are aware that circumstances have changed from the days when people endured months on orthopaedic wards, when, for example, a patient might be introduced to weaving or leatherwork as a way to maintain mental and physical health, and to provide some sense of purpose during the long period of confinement. Nevertheless, the loss of creative and productive occupations from the repertoire of occupational therapists has gone too far. Furthermore, it is proposed here that even the use of activities of daily living could benefit from a reconsideration of their creative potential, in order to enrich people's everyday experience.

This chapter introduces creativity, defines it and similar terms, and presents a theoretical stance that might help to justify the reintroduction of creative activities in occupational therapy in any setting. The chapter synthesizes recent knowledge and insights from occupational therapy, occupational science, neuroscience and the arts, to make a case for the return of creative occupations to practice. How and why occupational therapists have come to use many non-occupational interventions will be summarized from the literature. Consideration will be given to the idea that creativity could be a more central tenet of therapy. Efforts already made to bring creativity back will be outlined, and suggestions made regarding the wider use of creative occupations in practice.

7.2   Overview

The verb 'create' means to bring into being, into existence, to give rise to, to make by one's actions, or to manifest the un-manifest (*The Concise Oxford Dictionary*, 2002). It stems from the Latin *creare*, meaning 'to produce or generate' (*Word Power Dictionary*, 2001), and when applied to human life infers a high level activity. The adjective 'creative' is commonly used to suggest exceptional human ability, inventiveness, originality and imagination. Thus 'creativity' is the phenomenon of being able to create, while a 'creation' is defined as a 'product of human intelligence, especially creative thought' (*The Concise Oxford Dictionary*, 2002), which may not be material, but ephemeral, such as music and dance. However, creativity and related concepts can be interpreted more broadly to provide a new perspective on all levels of human activity.

The argument for restoring creativity to occupational therapy practice is essentially as follows. The hallmark of human beings is our evolution into a species with high level capacities, the pinnacle of which is creativity: the ability to change the material world to meet our needs and express ourselves through everyday activities, the arts, our interactions, and in fact, everything that we do. Wilcock (1998) has demonstrated that humans have a creative nature and to withhold or block that inherited ability is a denial of our true essence. Suppression of our potential can be seen as a stressor, which may lead to ill health, for example through the negative effects of stress on the immune system. Many people in society have had a long-term reduction in opportunities to express their creativity, which may contribute to their disease, or at least, to a reduced sense of well-being. If occupational therapists were more aware of these issues, we might be able to contribute more effectively to the well-being of those we serve, and to the health of societies everywhere.

7.2.1   Humans as creative beings

'*The key to our success is the possession of the most complex structure on Earth: the human brain*' (Suzuki, 1997, p. 9)

Occupational therapists can justify a return to using creative occupations by capitalizing on the growing understanding of creativity as a prime motivator of human occupation. Humans are seen as occupational beings; a species phylogenetically endowed with the capacity and need to participate in a wide range of creative occupations (Wood, 1993; Yerxa, 1998). Occupational science provides an insight into how the human physical form uniquely enables the enactment of creative expression. Wilcock's (1998) theory of the occupational nature of humans proposes that complex and unique occupational engagement is the destiny of the human species. She highlights how evolutionary factors such as bipedalism, skilled use of the hands, binocular vision, language and super consciousness have developed in innumerable combinations and permutations; testimony to human beings' creative intelligence and multiple ways of doing.

Occupational therapists would benefit from an increased awareness of other sciences, such as quantum physics which suggests that the universe is comprised only of energy. Even the composition of atomic particles such as electrons has been shown to be waves of energy, with no solid matter (Friedman, 1997). From this view, the form and function of the human species has evolved to the extent that each individual can be observed as a medium through which universal energy can bring about a metamorphosis of matter. Thus, a human being can take mud and turn it into a beautiful, more permanent object through the science of controlled fire and other manipulations of natural materials. In this way it is as if humans possess god-like abilities to create (Cameron, 1994). Humans have invented many methods of self-expression, which might be seen as the transformation of energy, including the musical, literary and visual arts. Human artistic creations have had a central place in our life experience throughout evolution. Indeed, made things become the evidence for early human habitation.

Creative activities usually provoke the senses, give pleasure and seem to help to connect to higher phenomena. The sounds of a choir or an orchestra, or the sight of a beautiful painting may elicit a feeling of spiritual connection through complex perceptions and emotions. Each art form has been refined to bring the utmost pleasure to one of the senses: such as music to hearing, painting to sight, literature to language. In order to achieve maximum stimulation, human senses demand high levels of complexity and symbolism. Creative occupations are an example of what humans can use to find and forge meaning in life (Trombly, 1995; White, 1996).

Creativity is associated with the spirit, in that humans create meaning in their lives through doing and making. The transcendental aspect of human experience has been brought into the centre of occupational therapy thinking through the Canadian Model of Occupational Performance (Law *et al.*, 1998) in particular, but is also included in other frameworks (e.g. Clark *et al.*, 1991). The spiritual aspect of creativity relates to the human need to connect and find a place in the world. Our super consciousness enables humans to see the connections between ourselves, others and the wider world. Humans have the potential to express or interpret these experiences, thoughts and feelings through artistic endeavours, such as material or ephemeral objects that enhance our world and provide new views of it. The human species seems to possess a creative energy which demands to be expressed, although that expression is often fraught with pain and anguish (Cameron, 1994). In seeking to understand the relationship between spirituality and human occupation, recent research into the brain and human intelligence is worth considering. Scientific developments have revealed that humans have three systems of intelligence: cognitive, emotional and spiritual (Zohar & Marshall, 2000).

Intellectual or rational intelligence relates to serial processing and logical thinking, and it relies on neural pathways similar to those responsible for reflexes, movement and sight. These pathways become hard wired through frequent repetition. The idea of hard wiring can be usefully deployed within occupational therapy for people with dementia, as habitual, manual skills may be retained after the decline of thinking and planning skills, enabling individuals to produce items which belie expectations (Josephsson, 1994).

Emotional intelligence, now called EQ, is that form of intelligence which enables us to feel emotions, and read them in others (Goleman, 1996). The neurones within this distinct associative network have many dendrites that form connections with thousands of others to contribute to holistic perceptions through a synthesis of the senses. In complex occupations, such as playing music, manual or oral skills become coordinated without conscious effort; emotional intelligence combines with intellectual intelligence to facilitate the higher interpretative judgement of responses and unique expressions of feeling that are the essence of art. Advances in brain imaging have led to the recent recognition of a third type of intelligence, spiritual intelligence, which manifests in oscillations of the brain rather than neural pathways. Spiritual intelligence is proposed to relate intimately with the kind of thinking that gives rise to intuition, insight, inventiveness, transcendence and finding meaning (Zohar & Marshall, 2000), and so is important to our understanding of creativity.

7.3   Creativity and current occupational therapy practice

It appears that the use of creative occupations in occupational therapy varies greatly depending on the setting and the country. In long-stay mental health units creative occupations may still have a place. The reduced use of creative occupations in physical and community settings, and the pre-eminence of functional assessments in many settings (Trombly, 1995), took hold during the seventh and eighth decades of the twentieth century. The reasons for this have been analysed in detail by Wilcock (1998) and include the strong influence of the medical model, a culture of prescription, medical patronage, the gender bias and reductionism. The almost extreme adaptability of the profession enabled therapists to fit well within almost any practice setting, often by adjusting to the environments where the prime concern was speedy throughput. Efforts to appear more professional and scientific contributed to the decline in creative and artistic pursuits, and an increase in the use of talking therapies such as group discussions, behavioural techniques and counselling. Anecdotal evidence suggests that many practising therapists vehemently reject the image of occupational therapy as being involved in creative activities, although this seems to be less the case in many mental health settings.

Another impediment to the use of creative activities, is that in everyday conversation creativity is associated with concepts such as the arts. However, Hasselkus (2002) helps us to take a wider interpretation, using theories within occupational therapy which pertain to creativity and occupation. She acknowledges that common perceptions associate creativity with exceptional accomplishments, like great achievements in the arts and sciences. However, if originality is seen as the key, even a mundane daily living activity can be performed in a creative manner, that is, it can be performed in a unique or unusual way. Pierce (2000) assists us further in this regard, by attempting to untangle the complex concepts of activity and occupation. She defines activity in contrast with other explanations (such as Hagedorn, 2001; Creek, 2003), where occupations are seen as the overarching term applied to the complex roles humans take, and activities are viewed as the component parts of these occupations.

Pierce (2000) proposes that the construct of activity should refer to the general ideas people hold about the things humans do, such as cooking. However, human beings have conscious will and so, by virtue of the volitional system, are able to modify, or even completely violate, the common understanding of how something is performed. It is this subjective experience of an individual performing an activity in his or her unique and never to be repeated way, which Pierce (2000) labels occupation. Construed in this way, occupation can be understood as the creative way an individual performs any activity. The uniqueness of occupational performance is valued by society, as is indicated by the worth attributed to originality in living styles, and also to works of artistic nature (White, 1996).

Viewing human occupation from this perspective may provide a useful way of understanding how humans use creativity to explore and find new ways of performing occupations in the face of illness, trauma or distress. People with disabilities, especially physical ones, gradually adapt through the invention of creative ways of doing everyday things such as getting dressed. It could be said that in these circumstances people create new occupational forms (Nelson, 1994). Occupational therapists should become partners in this creative undertaking, and to do so creativity needs to be widely interpreted in occupational therapy. Through occupation/activity analysis, a basic tool within occupational therapy, it can be demonstrated that virtually all human activities, even the most basic survival actions, have been raised to higher levels due to the human need and capacity for invention and expression in everything we do and make.

Our nutritional needs may serve as an illustration here. Compare, for example, the eating of natural vegetation, the method of sustaining the life force for many animal species, with humans participating in a special occasion dinner. In materially rich societies of today, the dinner table may be decorated with the best textiles, crockery and flowers. Careful attention is given to the seating arrangements and decoration of the room, to create the appropriate ambience, perhaps using background music and lighting effects. Each course of the meal is carefully planned, prepared and presented. Think also of the technology and science involved in making the ceramics and glassware that has taken thousands of years of human experience to perfect. It seems that humans need to create complex ways of performing even basic survival occupations, and that they can derive great pleasure from such experiences. The film *Babette's Feast* (Axel & Dinesen, 1988) is a powerful portrayal of the social healing and spiritual happiness that sharing a special meal can bring. It could be suggested then, that all survival skills have become arts or means for human expression: sheltering (external and internal architecture, home making), cleansing (bathroom rituals) and dressing (differential clothing, fashion).

We can thus make the connection that if creativity is essential to human well-being, then an absence of it can lead to ill health. One symptom of modern living is the reduced time spent on the occupation of preparing food and eating together, the negative results of which can only be imagined. Furthermore, the growing discontent and spiritual disconnection may be linked with a lack of experience in making beautiful things in this age of passive occupations such as watching television.

To recap, the theoretical position from the literature is this:

- The capacity to participate in creative activities is a major characteristic of our species.
- Engagement in creative occupations is linked to well-being.
- Non-participation in creative activities can precipitate ill health and disease due to the stress of not using given capacities.
- Creativity is a synthesis of intellectual, emotional and spiritual intelligence, and requires integration of the performance sub-systems.
- Human beings, through their creative potential, can elevate everything they do, including survival functions, to forms of art.
- Humans use their creativity to innovate and change the way they do things in an infinite variety of ways.
- As well as addressing items on a referral, a major aim of therapy should be to restore/enhance clients' creative capacities, for their own health's sake.

7.4   Creativity and future occupational therapy practice

Evidence-based approaches are vital to today's practice, and evidence is growing to support the observation that occupations are potent agents in health care. Hasselkus (1998) showed that when care workers involved a woman with severe dementia in flower arranging, which had been a long-term interest of hers, feelings of well-being were experienced by the client and her helpers. Moran and Strong (1995) found that involvement in a complex task may be more effective than prescribed medication in relieving pain. Mee and Sumsion (2001) showed that when people with long-term mental health problems participated in individual woodwork projects in a self-managed centre, their sense of well-being, motivation and self-worth was greatly enhanced. Older people report positive experiences in group activity programmes (Carlson *et al.*, 1996; Andersson-Sviden & Borell, 1998).

It is acknowledged that increases in material wealth in affluent Western countries have not brought comparative increased levels of happiness (Csikzentmihalyi, 1993; James, 1997). Instead, there has been an increase in mental illness (Wolpert, 1999) and so-called lifestyle diseases, such as coronary heart disease (Blaxter, 1990). The surge of applications in the UK for Voluntary Services Overseas perhaps indicates that more people seek life satisfaction and meaning through work rather than material gain (Voluntary Services Overseas, 2003).

Urban living, in particular, can lead to occupational alienation, when innate instincts and contact with the natural world are thwarted (Suzuki, 1997; Wilcock, 1998). People deprived of creative expression may then act negatively towards their own kind, or actually turn creative skills into destructive ones. The 'drifting dissatisfaction' of city life may be linked with vandalism and drug-related crime (Jenkins & Sherman, 1981, p. 5). The blocking of creativity is a form of what Wilcock (1998) has called occupational alienation: the prevention, through external conditions, from using one's full capacities. Vandalism may therefore be seen as a result of a creative nature not being nurtured. Issues of social exclusion, which may follow lack of a creative occupational role, are high on the political agenda in the UK. It seems that it is principally through occupations that human beings enact their chosen purpose in life and truly enjoy optimal experiences and conditions that are linked with a perception of well-being (Csikzentmihalyi, 1990, 1993). It is an issue of public health concern to occupational therapists that many people, in Western society at least, are not maximizing their creative potential, due to participation in too many pastimes that are essentially passive.

Human beings seem to have an instinctive drive to purposefully utilize creative occupations to relieve symptoms such as depression. Participants in a study by Reynolds (1998) revealed an intuitive need to relieve their agitation or depression through needlework projects of various types. One person created her designs during her 'high' periods, and literally stitched her way back up from times of feeling low. Another participant planned to embroider every species of owl for a museum, setting herself a lifelong task.

One major research study demonstrated that an occupational therapy programme, which included creative occupations for well elderly people, reduced the need for medical intervention and even hospitalization (Jackson *et al.*, 1998). In another large study it was found that participation in enjoyable occupations (such as card playing and dining out) impacted positively on the survival of elderly people at least as much as other known positive factors, such as exercise (Glass *et al.*, 1999).

These studies support the proposal that if a higher value was placed on returning creativity to occupational therapy, more therapists in all settings might have the courage to use these media. Occupational therapists might come to see creative occupational therapy methods through new eyes. This perspective allows us to appreciate that any occupation can be viewed as a creative act. Occupations are rarely simple, although others might see them as such. Occupational therapists could, for example, substitute clay for therapeutic putty in hand clinics; introduce poetry, drawing and creative writing to medical and surgical wards; refocus on gardening or embroidery during visits in the community; arrange for the creation of murals in youth detention centres. These changes are already starting to happen, and the possibilities are only limited by the creativity of the individual occupational therapist.

Another significant issue for the profession is that the teaching and use of creative arts and crafts as therapeutic media in occupational therapy training curricula has decreased. Ever-increasing pressure to make courses more academic, combined with the reduction in the use of creative media in the field, has led to dramatic reductions in the teaching of practical skills throughout the English-speaking areas of the world. Notably, this has not happened in Continental Europe, where many occupational therapy programmes retain strong creative activity experience for students (European Network of Occupational Therapists in Higher Education, 2002), although these seem to be under threat. If new graduates are not experienced or skilled in creative occupations they are not likely to use them in their practice. Other new creative therapies, such as art therapy, music therapy and dance therapy, are increasing in prominence, along with courses for activity organizers and diversional therapists. Other professions such as nursing, physiotherapy and psychology, are incorporating activities in their ways of working.

7.5 Future research

Creativity is greatly under-researched in occupational therapy but it has been given much more attention from other perspectives (Hasselkus, 2002). Identification of the actual process and expected outcomes of creative tasks is required. For example, how does choice/compulsion influence the effect of participating in creative occupations in treatment centres, and how do people view creative interventions? One aspect that must be addressed by the profession is the development of outcome measures for the health benefits of engagement in creative occupations. Another issue worthy of attention is children's engagement in creative occupations to higher levels (such as learning musical instruments, developing drawing skills) and its relationship with vandalism or drug use. Furthermore, do creative hobbies enhance well-being in older persons? Occupational science is raising awareness of the links between occupation and health in populations through highlighting relevant research from other disciplines. One way forward which is likely to be very productive is devising joint research projects where occupational therapists/occupational scientists work with artists and craftspeople to study the advantages of engagement in their crafts.

7.6 Conclusion

A case has been presented that human beings are by nature a creative species, and expression of that character is essential to health and feelings of satisfaction and well-being. For many reasons, creative activities have fallen off many occupational therapy practice and education agendas during the past thirty years. Now we seem to be returning to the wisdom of the founders, and attempting to substantiate this through research. There seems to be a new-found confidence in, and external validation of, the profession's original philosophy and values, such as the use of creative activities in assessment and treatment. It is proposed here that occupational therapists must recognize and value the creative nature of most occupations. We should view clinical practice as working with people to create new ways of doing everyday activities, creating new occupational forms. Occupational therapists should place higher value on how sensory and aesthetic needs raise the level of many daily activities to the realm of art. The ideas occupational therapists have always held now appear to have some important contributions to make to society.

The challenge is to believe that with each person with whom we work, the ultimate aim might be to realize their creative potential. If more people realized the connection between creativity and health, the well-being of humankind in general might be improved. If society is to gain maximum benefit from an occupational perspective of health, we need practitioners who possess a deep understanding of the complex issues of human occupation and within that, creativity. We require therapists who are able to collaborate with individuals, using not only professional skill and knowledge but also their own creativity. Therapists can draw on their own creativity to find ways of returning creative occupations to practice. This should not be too difficult as many occupational therapists are creative individuals, and many may have been attracted to the profession because of this apparent congruency. Reflection on our own participation in creative activities, combined with a deeper understanding of their therapeutic value, should support these changes. A particular challenge in this age of evidence-based practice is to identify specific therapeutic benefits of participation in creative occupations.

This aspect of health and social care requires confident, skilled and articulate occupational therapists who will be proactive in promoting health and quality of life through creative occupations, for all people. This message needs to reach out into the public domain. Just as the public are now more aware of the health effects of exercise, and of healthy eating, so too they should be conscious of the health benefits of exercising their creativity. Thus, if participation in creative occupations is the key which unlocks a sense of genuine well-being in our species, then maximizing humans' creative capacity should be our *raison d'être* in any setting.

References

Andersson-Sviden, G. & Borell, L. (1998). Phenomenon embedded in the experience of occupations – some elderly people's positive experiences of occupations included in community based activity programmes. *Scandinavian Journal of Occupational Therapy, 5*, 133–139.

Axel, G. & Dinesen, I. (Writers), G. Axel (Director) (1988). *Babette's Feast* (Motion picture). United States: Panorama.

Blaxter, M. (1990). *Health and Lifestyles*. London: Routledge.

Cameron, J. (1994). *The Artists' Way. A Course in Discovering and Recovering your Creative Self*. London: Pan Books.

Concise Oxford Dictionary (2002). Oxford: Oxford University Press.

Carlson, M., Fanchiang, S., Zemke, R. & Clark, F. (1996). A meta-analysis of the effectiveness of occupational therapy for older persons. *American Journal of Occupational Therapy, 50*, 89–98.

Clark, F., Parham, D., Carlson, M., Frank, G., Jackson, J., Pierce, D., Wolfe, R. & Zemke, R. (1991). Occupational science: academic innovation in the service of occupational therapy's future. *American Journal of Occupational Therapy, 45* (4), 300–310.

Creek, J. (2003). *Occupational Therapy Defined as a Complex Intervention.* London: College of Occupational Therapists.

Csikzentmihalyi, M. (1990). *Flow: the Psychology of Optimal Experience.* New York: Harper & Row.

Csikzentmihalyi, M. (1993). Activity and happiness: towards a science of occupation. *Journal of Occupational Science: Australia, 1* (1), 38–42.

European Network of Occupational Therapists in Higher Education (2002). *Teaching Practical Skills Project.* Amsterdam: European Network of Occupational Therapists in Higher Education.

Friedman, N. (1997). *The Hidden Domain. Home of Quantum Wave Function, Nature's Creative Source.* Woodbridge: Woodbridge Group.

Glass, T., De Leon, C., Marottoli, R. & Berkman, L. (1999). Population based study of social and productive activities as predictors of survival among elderly Americans. *British Medical Journal, 319,* 478–483.

Goleman, D. (1996). *Emotional Intelligence.* London: Bloomsbury.

Hagedorn, R. (2001). *Foundations for Practice in Occupational Therapy.* Edinburgh: Churchill Livingstone.

Hasselkus, B. (1998). Occupation and well-being in dementia: the experience of day-care staff. *American Journal of Occupational Therapy, 52* (6), 423–434.

Hasselkus, B. (2002). *The Meaning of Everyday Occupation.* Thorofare: Slack.

Jackson, J., Carlson, M., Mandel, D., Zemke, R. & Clark, F. (1998). Occupation in lifestyle redesign: the well elderly study occupational therapy programme. *American Journal of Occupational Therapy, 52* (5), 326–336.

James, O. (1997). *Britain on the Couch: Why We're Unhappier Compared with 1950, Despite Being Richer: a Treatment for the Low Serotonin Society.* London: Century.

Jenkins, C. & Sherman, B. (1981). *The Leisure Shock.* London: Eyre Methuen.

Josephsson, S. (1994). *Everyday Activities as Meeting Places in Dementia.* Stockholm: Krolinska Institute.

Law, M.C., Baptiste, S., Carswell, A., McColl, M.A., Polatajko, H. & Pollock, N. (1998). *The Canadian Occupational Performance Measure* (3rd Edn). Toronto: Canadian Association of Occupational Therapists.

Mee, J. & Sumsion, T. (2001) Mental health clients confirm the motivating power of occupation. *British Journal of Occupational Therapy, 64* (3), 121–128.

Moran, M. & Strong, J. (1995). Outcomes of a rehabilitation programme for patients with chronic back pain. *British Journal of Occupational Therapy, 58* (19), 435–458.

Nelson, D. (1994). Occupational form, occupational performance, and therapeutic occupation. In: C. Royeen (Ed.), *The Practice of the Future: Putting Occupation Back into Therapy.* Rockville, Md.: American Occupational Therapy Association.

Pierce, D. (2000). Untangling occupation and activity. *American Journal of Occupational Therapy, 55,* 138–146.

Reynolds, F. (1998). Needlework in the Management of Anxiety and Depression. Paper presented at the College of Occupational Therapists' Annual Conference, Belfast.

Suzuki, D. (1997). *The Sacred Balance. Rediscovering our Place in Nature.* Vancouver: Greystone Books.

Trombly, C. (1995). Occupation: purposefulness and meaningfulness as therapeutic mechanisms. *American Journal of Occupational Therapy, 49,* 960–972.

Voluntary Services Overseas (2003). *The Meaning of Work.* Retrieved 24 September, 2003, from: www.one world.org/vso/news/meaning.htm

White, J. (1996). Miles Davis: Occupations in the extreme. In: R. Zemke & F. Clark (Eds), *Occupational Science: the Evolving Discipline* (pp. 259–273). Philadelphia: F.A. Davis.

Wilcock, A. (1998). *An Occupational Perspective of Health.* Thorofare: Slack.

Wolpert, L. (1999). *Malignant Sadness: the Anatomy of Depression.* London: Faber & Faber.

Wood, W. (1993). Occupation and the relevance of primatology to occupational therapy. *American Journal of Occupational Therapy, 47* (6), 515–522.

Word Power Dictionary (2001). Pleasantville: Readers' Digest.

Yerxa, E. (1998). Health and the human spirit for occupation. *American Journal of Occupational Therapy, 52* (6), 412–418.

Zohar, D. & Marshall, I. (2000). *SQ. Spiritual Intelligence.* Edinburgh: Bloomsbury.

Section B
Practising in an Occupational Way

Chapter 8
Occupational Performance Issues in Pretend Play: Implications for Paediatric Practice

Karen Stagnitti

Two healthy four year-old boys were playing in a sandpit. One of the boys, Tom, hit a tin repeatedly with a stick, then placed the stick in the tin and then resumed using the stick to hit the tin. In between hitting the tin with the stick he would put sand in the tin and then tip the sand out into the sandpit. The activity was repeated until he was interrupted by an adult who invited Tom to have a swing. Tom left with the adult. After examining the now abandoned tin and stick, the other four year-old, Greg, placed the stick across the tin and lifted it into the air making an engine noise. The 'plane' then came in to land. While the engine noises continued with an 'engine running' type sound, Greg placed sand into the tin and lifted the 'plane' into the air with 'taking-off' engine noises. The 'plane' was brought in to land on the other side of the sandpit and the sand was emptied methodically from the 'plane'. Greg then used the tin and stick as a bulldozer and made a maze of roads. A third child noticed Greg playing and came to ask if he could join in with the play. The two children then continued the theme of transport vehicles by adding bridges, tunnels and water holes to the play scene in the sandpit.

8.1   Introduction

Occupational therapists working within paediatrics are concerned with daily life activities of the child that have meaning to the child (Humphry, 2002). These daily life activities are the child's occupations, and play is regarded as the primary occupation of childhood (Canadian Association of Occupational Therapists, 1996). In this chapter the view is taken that play is valuable in and of itself, and that the occupational performance of play impacts on a child's functioning in society. 'Play ... may be understood as a vehicle of meaning ... Thus from this perspective, play becomes a quality of life issue in the here and now' (Parham & Primeau, 1997, p. 17). The opening story describes two children who have differences in their occupational performance of play. The differences in the play of these two children is examined in this chapter and related to the child's participation in society. As preparation for this discussion the concept of play is examined. This is followed by a discussion of the value of play to child development. The chapter is concluded by a case study that is taken from clinical practice. In the case study, the occupational assessment and treatment of play is described.

8.2   Overview: the concept of play

The understanding that play is important in itself, is an occupation that has meaning for the child and is the primary occupation of childhood, is a recent development in occupational therapy (Parham & Primeau, 1997; Rodger & Ziviani, 1999). For many years, occupational therapists viewed play behaviour as secondary to learning and therefore unscientific, with many occupational therapists embarrassed by being called 'play ladies' (Robinson, 1977; Bundy, 1991, 1997, 2001; Parham & Primeau, 1997). Hence, many occupational therapists placed greater emphasis on non-play skill development such as motor skills (Couch *et al.*, 1997). The emphasis on non-play skill development represented a fundamental change in the practice of paediatric occupational therapy because play was no longer assessed or treated (Couch *et al.*, 1997; Parham & Primeau, 1997). One of the reasons for the avoidance of play in occupational therapy was a lack of understanding of play as a meaningful occupation for the child.

Under the leadership of Mary Reilly, play was given a place of importance in occupational therapy theory as a child's occupation (Reilly, 1974a; Parham & Primeau, 1997). Reilly's approach to play was influenced by many different viewpoints. However, the arousal modulation theories of play were highly influential in her view of play. These theories proposed that play behaviour was maintained by the curiosity of the child and the child's exploration of objects, and that through play the child prepared for adaptation to adult life. The functionalist view of play, which proposes that play is a means to develop other skills, justifies the use of play in the clinical situation but it does not recognize that play is legitimate in itself (Parham & Primeau, 1997).

The understanding of play as occupation has been interpreted in the broadest of terms in occupational therapy. For example, play is regarded as an all encompassing activity which helps develop skills in cognition, socialization, communication, self-awareness, problem solving, and sensorimotor functions (Canadian Association of Occupational Therapists, 1996). Play is believed to facilitate flexibility in thinking, adaptability, learning, problem solving, exploration to gain a sense of mastery over one's environment, information integration from the environment, and development of social, intellectual, emotional and physical skills (Michelman, 1974; Howard, 1986; von Zuben *et al.*, 1991; Canadian Association of Occupational Therapists, 1996). Play is also believed to facilitate integration, survival and an understanding of a culture (Vandenberg & Kielhofner, 1982).

In practice, these broad views of play have resulted in occupational therapists not prioritizing play assessment and play treatment because play is not operationally defined (Bundy, 1991, 1993; Parham & Primeau, 1997). Surveys of assessments used in occupational therapy either do not list play assessments as important in practice or do not list assessments of play at all (Reid, 1987; Rodger, 1994; Couch *et al.*, 1997). As a consequence of not assessing play, many occupational therapists use play in a secondary role as a means to gain observations and improvements in skills such as attention, motor skills and sensory processing (Rodger & Ziviani, 1999; Stagnitti *et al.*, 2000).

For play to be regarded as valuable in itself, a clearer understanding of play is needed. This is not an easy task as play is a complex behaviour that appears deceptively simple (Knox, 1974; Reilly, 1974b; Robinson, 1977; de Renne-Stephan, 1980; von Zuben *et al.*, 1991). The practical result of the complexity of play is that it is difficult to define as a distinct behaviour. However, in an effort to address this problem researchers in occupational therapy and other disciplines have concluded that play (Stewart *et al.*, 1991; Bracegirdle, 1992; Goodman, 1994; Bundy, 1997; Parham & Primeau, 1997):

- Is more internally than externally motivated
- Transcends reality as well as reflects reality
- Is controlled by the player
- Involves more attention to process than product
- Is safe
- Is usually fun, unpredictable, pleasurable
- Is spontaneous and involves non-obligatory active engagement

Play has also been defined as exploratory in nature, and consisting of a variety of activities that involve movement and manipulation in relation to the environment (Robinson, 1977).

8.2.1 Re-examining play – play has value in itself

Since play is difficult to define, it is difficult to assess and so the occupational performance of play is rarely addressed in clinical practice. The non-clinical assessment of play is compounded because occupational therapy play assessments that are available assess the child in his/her familiar environment (e.g. Knox, 1974; The Preschool Play Scale, Bledsoe & Shepherd, 1982; Test of Playfulness, Bundy, 2001).

To be able to assess play in a clinical setting, the concept of play has to be re-examined from the view that play has unique value in itself and can be distinguished from other behaviours. In the opening story of the two four-year-old boys playing in the sandpit, one child used symbols in play (i.e. the tin and stick represented a plane) whereas the other child manipulated and explored the objects. There is a major distinction in the play of these two children. The use of symbols in play has been called symbolic play and when children use symbols in play there is always an element of pretence. When children pretend there is no doubt that they are playing. For example, Cross and Coster (1997, p. 810) noted that the use of symbolic play language 'does highlight whether and when play is happening'. Cognitive developmental theorists assume that play involves the use of symbols and that play is distinguished from other general forms of activity by the creation of imaginary situations (e.g. Vygotsky, 1966). The cognitive developmental theorists of play understood play as being pretend play. Pretend play is regarded as the mature form of play for the pre-schooler and the most challenging form of play for the child (Vygotsky, 1966, 1997). In this respect, pretend play has meaning for the child because it is interesting, challenging and gives the child a quality of life in terms of social communication with peers, practice in using language and development of abstract thought. Pretend play is an occupation of childhood.

While the occupational therapy profession has included aspects of cognitive developmental theories of play in its view of play, pretend play *per se* has not been recognized as valuable in itself. Pretend play has been used as a means to an end in occupational therapy (i.e. using pretend play as a motivation in therapy to develop other skills). Using pretend play as a means to an end results in non-identification of play behaviour that is significant to cognitive, social and language development. For example, during sensory integration therapy, symbolic play language (symbolic play is an aspect of pretend play) is used frequently by the child and the therapist (Cross & Coster, 1997). Thus, a child might pretend that the bolster swing is a bull (Bundy, 1991). Cross and Coster (1997) reported that symbolic play language was used as a method to engage children in sensory integration activities. The use of pretend play in this manner does not recognize the occupational value of pretend play because pretend play is used as a means to maintain the child's attention, concentration and enjoyment of the therapy.

8.2.2   Defining pretend play

Pretend play is important in a child's development, and pre-school children spend a lot of time and energy engaged in the occupation of pretending in play. For example, by 48 months of age children spend 'an average of 12.4 minutes per hour pretending' (Haight & Miller, 1993, p. 118). To help understand pretend play it is defined below in a precise manner. Pretend play includes both symbolic play and conventional imaginative play. Lewis *et al.* (1992) defined symbolic play as play involving substitution of one object to represent another; the attribution of a property to an action or object (e.g. the box 'oven' is hot); and reference to an absent object (e.g. the wave of an arm represents a doorway). For these to occur, the child is required to transcend reality. For example, when a child pretends a shoe is a train, the reality of the shoe is suspended while the child 'drives' the shoe. Symbolic play is most easily seen in play when the child uses an object (e.g. a stick or a shoe) in an unconventional way by pretending the object is something else.

The conventional use of objects, such as placing a doll in a bed, is regarded as conventional imaginative play. Conventional imaginative play occurs when the child uses conventional toys to pretend. With conventional toys the child can put a doll in a bed and pretend the doll is asleep or fill up a truck with 'petrol'. Conventional imaginative play is play that reflects reality. Some authors refer to conventional imaginative play as 'functional play' because the child relates the objects functionally, for example, the chair is placed at the table (Casby, 1992; Lewis & Boucher, 1997). However, the attributes of symbolic play can also be observed in conventional imaginative play (Stagnitti & Unsworth, 2000). For example, a hat can be used for a boat (object substitution), a doll can be sick (property attribution) and a wave of the arm can refer to a door (reference to an absent object).

The above definition of pretend play assumes that the child can self-initiate pretend play, that is, it is spontaneous. By including both symbolic play and conventional imaginative play in the definition of pretend play, the child's ability to substitute objects, attribute properties to objects and refer to absent objects is acknowledged to occur in play with both conventional toys and objects. By specifying the attributes of pretend play behaviour it is possible to distinguish pretend play from other play behaviours such as exploration, running and manipulation. In the opening story of the two boys playing, it can now be seen that the occupational performance in pretend play was the difference between the play behaviour of the two boys. Tom's play was exploratory. He hit the tin with the stick, he put sand in the tin and poured it out. Greg played with the same objects as Tom, but he used the objects as symbols. The tin and stick became a plane. Greg then used the 'plane' he had made in a series of actions which developed into a story. The result of this was that another child came to join Greg in play. The occupational performance in pretend play of both boys had meaning for them and provided a common basis to participate together in play.

Pretend play as occupation

Pretend play develops in the second year of life. Before the appearance of pretend play, play takes the form of exploration and manipulation. Many skills, which are foundation skills for further play development, are mastered during the first two years of life such as manipulation, object permanence and imitation (McCune Nicolich, 1977; Pierce, 1997; Stagnitti, 1998). The child's ability to explore and manipulate objects extends beyond the second year of life and is important throughout life. However, between the ages of eighteen months to seven years pretend play is the most challenging and mature form of play. After seven years of age play changes in form, although the skills learnt through pretend in play are utilized throughout life. For example, as a result of the ability to pretend play, people understand non-literal concepts and situations. Pretend play is important to the social, cognitive and communication development of the individual. Pretend play then, can be viewed from the functionalist position as well as the position that it is valuable in itself and has meaning to the child.

Using the World Health Organization's *International Classification of Functioning* (ICF) (WHO, 2001), Stagnitti and Unsworth (2000) illustrated the connection between skills needed for pretend play, occupation in pretend play and participation in social situations. Stagnitti and Unsworth argued that the child's occupational performance in pretend play assisted the child to participate in society as a player. The occupational performance components that are required for a child to pretend play include cognitive, emotional and social aspects. If there are impairments in any of these components then the child presents with occupational limitations in pretend play. It is proposed that occupational limitations in pretend play lead to restricted participation in society, which has social, emotional and cognitive (or learning) consequences for the child.

The cognitive skills that are required for occupational performance of pretend play include those skills that have been linked with literacy, such as narrative competence, organization of thinking, decontextualized language ability (i.e. use of language 'out of context', such as using language associated with spaceships when the child is sitting in a box), and representing thoughts in writing (Schrader, 1989; Pellegrini & Galda, 1993). Attention, concentration, memory and visualization are important to the duration of time a child spends in play and are included as cognitive capacities involved in pretend play. Children often pretend in play with other children. Through playing out life's social roles, the child becomes aware of the norms and rules of behaviour; for example, playing 'mothers' reflects rules of maternal behaviour (Vygotsky, 1966). Pretend play enables the child to act out situations with different outcomes to reality (Vygotsky, 1966). The ability to pretend during play enables the capacity to decentre from the self by giving objects characteristics and motives, and this develops in the child an ability to understand the perspective of others (Rubin *et al.*, 1983; Baron-Cohen, 1996).

Westby (1991) noted that pretend play affects all areas of development and facilitates the healthy development of emotions, convergent and divergent thought, language-literacy, impulse control, perspective taking and socialization. In summary, pretend play is important in child development because it:

- Encompasses and reflects important cognitive skills in the development of the child (Piaget, 1962; Fein, 1975; Ungerer *et al.*, 1981; Sparling *et al.*, 1984; Power & Radcliffe, 1991; Pellegrini & Galda, 1993; Wyver & Spence, 1995).
- Is important to language development (Westby, 1991; Lewis *et al.*, 2000).
- Heralds the beginning of theory of mind and consequently social perceptiveness (Baron-Cohen, 1996).
- Is important to emotional development (Vygotsky, 1966).
- Is the primary occupation of childhood because it has meaning for the child.

A child's motor and sensory skills are listed as components that support pretend play because these skills enable a child to manipulate objects (Stagnitti & Unsworth, 2000). However, manipulation of objects is given a minor role as manipulation and exploration of objects is a primary form of play that occurs during the first 18 months of life (Stagnitti & Unsworth, 2000).

By observing children in play, the importance of the occupation of pretend play becomes clear. Reflect back to the two children described in the opening of this chapter. Greg was typically developing in his pretend play ability, and the occupational performance components of his play that were important to the occupation of pretend play are listed in Table 8.1, where they are contrasted with Tom's occupational performance in pretend play. Greg's occupational performance in pretend play enabled him to spontaneously participate with another peer in play. Tom did not participate in play with his peers; instead he interacted with objects in social isolation.

Table 8.1   A comparison of the occupational performance of Tom and Greg's pretend play.

Tom	Greg
• He did not use symbols in play.	• He was able to use objects as symbols in play.
• His play was repetitive.	
• He did not initiate play ideas but rather repeated exploratory play behaviour.	• He was flexible in adjusting to other's ideas in play and thus adapted to another child joining him in play.
• His peers did not join him in his play.	
• He could not sustain a play scenario over a period of time.	• He was able to sustain and elaborate a play situation because he was able to logically sequence his play actions and thus his play developed into a story about transport vehicles (i.e. narrative competence was being developed).
• He did not extend his play by developing new play ideas.	
• There was no 'story', narrative or logical sequential play actions evidenced in his play.	
• There were no play themes in this play.	• A play theme was evident in Greg's play.
• There was no evidence of pretence in his play.	• He was able to negotiate and include other children in play.
• He required adult intervention to change the activity.	• He was able to self-initiate his own play.

Assessing the occupational performance of pretend play

The understanding of pretend play as occupational performance and valuable in itself has resulted in the development of the Child-Initiated Pretend Play Assessment (ChIPPA) (Stagnitti, 2002). The ChIPPA was developed based on the assumptions that play is measurable and valuable in itself and that there are unique attributes of play behaviour that are always present and essential to play. The ChIPPA is a 30-minute norm-referenced standardized assessment that can be used in a clinical situation. The ChIPPA measures a child's spontaneous pretend play ability by assessing their conventional imaginative play and symbolic play in the same assessment session. In this way play is measured as a dynamic, fluid activity. Three play attributes are measured on the ChIPPA. These are: the child's elaborate pretend play actions (i.e. play actions that are used in a sequence to develop a story or construction), the child's ability to substitute objects (i.e. use symbols in play), and the child's reliance on a model to play (i.e. the number of times the child imitates the examiner).

A child's elaborate play raw scores in the conventional imaginative play session and symbolic play session, and a child's raw scores relating to object substitution in the symbolic play session can be compared to z scores for his or her age group. Z scores indicate what is normal range and whether children need interventions or not (interventions indicated by scores of -2 or more). For the scores relating to use of objects with the conventional imaginative play session and the scores for the imitated actions for both sessions of the ChIPPA, the child's raw score is compared to the mode, as typical children score 0 for these items. These quantitative scores are considered alongside qualitative information of the child's pretend play that is gathered on the ChIPPA clinical observations form.

The most common play profile on the ChIPPA for typically developing children is within normal range or higher for all elaborate pretend play actions and within normal range or higher for object substitutions in the symbolic play session. Typical children do not need a model to develop play ideas and therefore they do not imitate the examiner (scoring 0), and they mostly use the conventional toys in conventional ways, thus scoring 0 for object substitutions with conventional imaginative play. The ChIPPA identifies play dysfunction and interprets this dysfunction with respect to a child's development and ability to learn.

The quantitative and qualitative information gathered on the ChIPPA is used in conjunction with the parent or carer's observations and concerns of the child's play to identify a child's strengths and resources, the occupational performance components of pretend play, and any relevant environmental conditions. This allows for further clarification of issues relating to the child's pretend play occupation such as occupational deprivation (e.g. lack of play ability or opportunity), occupational justice (e.g. the child's play needs are not met due to circumstances) and alienation (e.g. the child only plays with one type of toy, such as a truck, to the exclusion of all else). When the ChIPPA is used in conjunction with a battery of assessments (e.g. developmental, motor and visual perceptual assessment), issues of occupational imbalance can also be identified (e.g. the child spends all his/her time in activities of daily living and no time is left for play).

Since the ChIPPA is an assessment of the occupational performance of pretend play, it enables an occupational approach to treatment through the Learn to Play programme (Stagnitti, 1998). This treatment approach uses pretend play as the intervention to improve a child's occupation in play. As Parham and Primeau (1997) noted, the 'acknowledgment that play is important in its own right opens the door to intervention that makes enhancement of the child's play life the goal' (p. 18). The way in which a child's play is assessed and treated as the primary occupation in childhood is illustrated in the case study below.

8.3   John: a case study

8.3.1   Referral

'John' was referred to an occupational therapy clinic in a government run community based early intervention service at the age of two years because his mother had concerns about his development. He had undergone one operation to correct a hip displacement and this had resulted in hip spica plasters being applied to his legs for six months in the first two years of his life. As well as medical and developmental concerns, John's mother 'Jenny' suspected that he had autism spectrum disorder because he displayed flapping movements of his hands, gave poor eye contact, did not seem interested in people and loved to look at lights. An assessment for autism was organized at the age of two years and the conclusion was reached that John was not autistic. A developmental assessment at two years of age, using the Hawaii Early Learning Profile (VORT Corporation, 1995), revealed that John presented with sensorimotor problems. His fine motor ability was excellent for his age, but his gross motor skills were delayed. For example, John did not walk until two years of age and this was directly related to his hip spica plasters. His cognitive skills were scattered, and self-care skills were delayed due to the fact that he was very passive. John did not show an interest in social situations. He was more excited by cars and bikes than he was by meeting familiar people. Alienation was apparent in his play as, for example, he loved wheels, buses and cars to the exclusion of all other play materials. He would stare out of the window for long periods of time looking at leaves flapping in the wind and cars driving past. He did not demand attention and was happy to lie in his bed and gaze at the ceiling. A home programme was implemented based on sensorimotor activities.

At the age of four years, Jenny was still concerned that John was autistic. As he had grown, his parents had noted that: he would only accept the same cereal for breakfast each morning, he liked any object that was yellow, he was rigid in his social interactions, and his play was limited. He was referred again to a specialist service for an assessment for autism spectrum disorder. On assessment by the specialist service John was diagnosed with autism spectrum disorder.

8.3.2 Assessment of John's occupational difficulties

A reassessment of his development showed that John had poor sensory modulation and his balance was reduced. A speech therapy assessment reported that his language was delayed. At this time John's play was assessed using the newly developed Child-Initiated Pretend Play Assessment (ChIPPA) (Stagnitti, 2002). Compared to typically developing children also aged four years one month, John's ChIPPA results indicated that his ability to sequence play actions was below normal age range. He could use symbols in play, his play with conventional toys was more delayed than his play with unstructured objects, and he found it difficult to initiate and extend play ideas and themes. His results are detailed in Table 8.2.

Children who have occupational performance difficulties in pretend play often have difficulty playing with their peers, and social communication skills are at risk. The clinical observations noted during his ChIPPA assessment indicated that John could not concentrate for the time needed to complete the assessment,

Table 8.2 John's Child-Initiated Pretend Play Assessment results at age 4 years 1 month

ChIPPA play measure	Result	Interpretation of result
PEPA conventional	−3.29	Significant delay with John being outside 95% of children in the typical sample. This result is equivalent to below 1% if percentile ranks were used.
PEPA symbolic	−0.64	Within normal limits for his age.
PEPA combined	−2.00	Total elaborate play score which indicates that John's play ability is significantly delayed. This score is equivalent to the 2nd percentile.
NOS conventional	1	The mode for this score is 0 as most children use the conventional toys in a conventional manner. This score indicates that John can use symbols in play.
NOS symbolic	−0.44	John is able to use symbols in play. This result is within normal range for his age.
NOS combined	−0.22	This result is within normal range for his age.
NIA conventional	1	The mode for this score is 0 as most typically developing children do not imitate the examiner as they do not need a model to play. A score of 1 is still within normal range.
NIA symbolic	1	The mode for this score is 0 as most typically developing children do not imitate the examiner as they do not need a model to play. A score of 1 is still within normal range.
NIA combined	2	The mode for this score is 0 as most typically developing children do not imitate the examiner as they do not need a model of play. A score of 2 is still within normal range of 0–2.

Key: PEPA: percentage of elaborate pretend play actions: NOS: number of object substitutions; NIA: number of imitated actions; Conventional: the scores relate to the conventional imaginative play session of the ChIPPA; Symbolic: the scores relate to the symbolic play session of the ChIPPA; Combined: the scores relate to the conventional imaginative play session plus the symbolic play session of the ChIPPA

denoting that he could not sustain a play session. Other occupational performance issues were: not being able to extend his play, no use of narrative development during play, not talking about his play as he played and the doll was ignored during play.

As well as the ChIPPA assessment, other observations were made of John's abilities at the local early intervention playgroup. In this setting it was observed that John would not sit on the mat for a story or a singing session. He screamed each time he attended, did not interact with the other children, and was obsessed with all the yellow toys in the room and would not share them with other children. At home, John often fought with his siblings, he was rigid in his play ideas and this made his siblings frustrated and angry. He would ruin the play of his older sister by not cooperating in her pretend play scenarios.

8.3.3 Planning the occupational therapy intervention

Analysis of assessment findings identified the occupational performance components and environmental conditions contributing to John's difficulties. These were:

- Poor sensory modulation
- Reduced ability in balance
- Delayed sequencing of play actions, particularly in conventional-imaginative play
- Difficulty sustaining and extending a play idea
- Inability to play with others
- Delayed language

His parents identified occupational performance issues as:

- Becoming overexcited
- Fighting with siblings

The strengths and resources available to John were:

- A supportive home environment
- Involvement in an early childhood intervention playgroup
- Supportive social network of the family
- The therapist's experience

Outcomes were negotiated with the parents and it was decided to pursue intervention using sensorimotor techniques to gain a reduction in John's reactions to the sensory/environmental inputs. After six weeks this outcome was reassessed with John's parents. Even though calming techniques had been used in every session and John's parents had implemented calming techniques at home, John was still overreacting to sensory and environmental input and no follow-through had been noted in the home environment. Occupational performance issues were reconsidered with John's parents and it was decided that his occupational performance in pretend play (which included alienation in type of toys used, restricted ability to play with his siblings and peers and the consequent social isolation) were priority issues for John and his parents. The agreed plan was for John to be seen fortnightly at home using the Learn to Play programme and his parents were shown how to enable play in everyday life at home.

8.3.4 Implementing the occupational therapy intervention

The Learn to Play programme is a dynamic, interactive, play training programme. The term 'play training' is used to distinguish it from play therapy. Play therapy has evolved from the psychodynamic theories of play with play therapy used in child psychiatry clinics. Play training, by contrast, has its origins in the cognitive developmental theories of play and is based on the typical development of pretend play ability. Learn to Play has as the central principle that occupational performance in pretend play is essential for a child to fulfil the role of player thus enabling participation in society. The programme begins on the child's develop-mental pretend play level (not chronological age), and from this starting point play activities involving play themes, sequences of play actions, object substitu-tion, role play, social interaction and doll/teddy play are modelled for the child. Using the Learn to Play programme, the child is enabled to play by encouraging them to attend to the toys being used, modelling of the play activity by the therapist or parent, repeating the activity at least three times and talking about what is being played. The child is encouraged to join in with the play. Alienation or rote learning of play skills is avoided by generalizing the ability level being focused upon through different toys and play scenes that are on the same developmental level. For example, the use of symbols in play is an object sub-stitution ability. On the 20-month level the child develops the ability to use the same object for two different functions such as using a box for a table and a car in the same play session. This object substitution ability level is reinforced by also using a yellow block for hay for a cow and then as soap for a doll. The principle of the Learn to Play programme is to enable the child to initiate their own play ideas. Therefore, the child is encouraged to join in the play and as they become able to participate the therapist models less and follows the child's ideas in the play. For children with autism spectrum disorder, emphasizing the emotional interaction during pretend play is essential so that they can fully benefit from play training (Sherratt, 2002). As children become competent in occupational performance at the current developmental level of pretend play, the play skills on the next developmental level of pretend play are introduced into the sessions.

Play training activities for John began on the 18-month level for sequences in play action. That is, intervention began by using only one action in a play scene. For example, the teddy was given a cup to have to 'drink'. In the first sessions, particularly when the developmental level begins at 18 months, the therapist needs to prepare at least five play scenarios or scenes for the session. For example, the five play scenes may include feeding the teddy, placing the teddy in a car and going for a ride, feeding a doll, using a block train to take the teddy for a ride and stirring a pot for cooking. Each play scene is repeated and modelled at least three times and after each play scene the child is given a break. John's parents also took opportunities at home to reinforce the occupational performance in pretend play that was being addressed in therapy.

After three months of play training John could be involved in play activities that involved four or five play actions, indicating that the complexity of his play was developing. He could extend his object substitution skills to include less realistic objects, he could extend repetitive play themes by adding original ideas to the play sequence and he was beginning to include imaginary objects in play. He had just begun to spontaneously initiate the next play action in a sequence. Also at this time, several improvements were noted in his participation with others in play. He no longer destroyed his sister's pretend play scenes, but would let her direct him in the play. It is proposed that John now had the concept that something was happening even though he did not fully understand it. He had greater understanding of the social situation in the sandpit at the early intervention group and he would allow other children to use the yellow toys and wait for his turn. John was greeting people more appropriately and was understanding turn taking in different social situations.

After six months of play training, John had begun pre-school. His teacher noted that he did not join in with group play, he found it difficult to sit on the mat for mat time, he still preferred yellow toys and he did not easily share with others. Play training sessions continued at home on a fortnightly basis and his parents and pre-school teacher provided opportunities for pretend play in the home and pre-school environment, respectively. During this time John was challenged in his play skills to reach the three-year level. Play scenes during this time used several sequences, for example, a doll 'walked up a mountain', fell down and hurt its leg, the ambulance came and the doll was placed in a hospital bed while its leg was wrapped with a bandage. When the doll was well again, the doll would walk out of the hospital. Other play scenes also included pretending to post letters to different dolls' houses. For example, letters would be written and placed in the postbox. John would then empty the postbox into a post satchel and then, with modelling from the therapist, the letters would be delivered to different dolls' houses (usually chairs), and the dolls would read their letters 'excitedly'. Modelling by the therapist during this time also targeted the emotional aspects of playing with the doll as a character. For example, the doll was happy, the doll was sad. John did not seem to understand the emotional intent and pretended to throw the doll in the rubbish bin, laughing as he did it.

John's play training sessions continued. Seven months into John's pre-school year, and after 15 months of fortnightly play training John's play skills were now at a four-year level. This involved only two play scenes per play training session with several sequential actions used in play narratives, use of objects on an abstract level, characterization of the doll and play themes that included sub-plots in the story. In one such session the therapist took along some adult shoes and as these were tipped out on the floor, the therapist said that this was the new train set for the session. John's play skills were now on the developmental level where he understood that objects with their own meaning could be used as something else in play. Thus, using the shoes as a train posed no problems. The play theme revolved around dolls having a train ride and stopping at several destinations during the play scenes. Thus, John's sequences in play actions were longer and this resulted in longer storylines during the play and an extension of the time spent in play.

When John began to play more spontaneously on this level during play training sessions, his pre-school teacher noted some significant changes. Notably, for the first time John spent one hour in the sandpit in cooperative group play with four other children pretending there were roads, bridges and transport vehicles working together. He was now more flexible in accepting changes to his play and was more tolerant of changes made by others during the play. During this time his father recounted an event when he and John were walking by a river close to their home. John had noticed a plastic bag in the river and he began to tell his father how the plastic got there, what it was doing and where it was going. John was developing narrative – logical sequential thought with a pretend element and the ability to understand what would happen next.

As the year progressed, John was encouraged to engage in play themes on the five-year level, playing pirates and other themes that he had not personally experienced. He enjoyed these sessions and it was noted in play training sessions that he was now leading the play, adding new sequences to the play story, pretending there were 'bad' pirates that were watching and using several objects during play to represent other objects. During this time, he began to use the dolls as characters and carefully placed dolls in a scene. For example, he would place them carefully at a 'shoebox' table, or place a spherical shape at their feet to play football. At pre-school he was now playing with groups of children on a regular basis. For example, one girl at his pre-school had flown to London for a holiday and when she came back to pre-school she wanted to play 'flying to London'. With no direction from the teacher, the children spontaneously created the inside of an aeroplane by setting up rows of seats, an aisle made from mats, little boxes of 'food', a toilet area and earphones to listen to music while they were on the 'flight'. In this play setting, John's occupational performance in pretend play was commensurate with his peers, as he was the air steward and was responsible for handing out the food. He had an enjoyable time playing with the other children. He was participating with his peers as a player.

8.3.5   Evaluation and discharge

At the age of five years six months, John was reassessed on the ChIPPA and his scores were compared to a normative sample for his age. His results, presented in Table 8.3, showed that his occupational performance in pretend play had improved in most areas, particularly in his ability to play with conventional toys. He no longer showed alienation because he could now play with conventional toys as well as with unstructured objects. Clinical observations noted that John could attend to the play sessions for the total time of the assessment: he used the doll during play, he could develop narrative, he was more organized and he could extend his play. He was more cooperative in play with his siblings. In negotiation with John's parents play training sessions ceased, as John's improvement in his occupational performance of pretend play and his participation in play with his peers had greatly improved.

John began school the year following his pre-school year. His schoolteacher noted that he had good imagination, he contributed at mat time by answering questions about the story being read, he contributed to class discussion and he could follow what was required of him in the classroom. At lunch time he played in the sandpit with the other children without incident. John could follow a conversation and contribute to a conversation as well as initiating appropriate conversations with others. John enjoyed school and he enjoyed life. At home, while there were still fights between siblings, there was also time spent playing with siblings. For example, John has been observed recreating a television lifestyle

Table 8.3 John's Child-Initiated Pretend Play Assessment results at age 5 years 6 months

ChIPPA play measure	Result	Interpretation of result
PEPA conventional	−1.85 (−3.29)*	This score indicates that John's pretend play with conventional toys is delayed but is now within 95% of typical children.
PEPA symbolic	−0.60 (−0.64)*	Within normal limits for his age.
PEPA combined	−1.33 (−2.00)*	Overall score indicates that John's play ability is delayed but that it is now within 95% of the scores of typical children.
NOS conventional	2 (1)*	The mode for this score is 0 as most children use the conventional toys in a conventional manner. This score indicates that John can use symbols in play and that he has improved since initial assessment.
NOS symbolic	−0.40 (−0.44)*	John is able to use symbols in play. This result is within normal range for his age.
NOS combined	−0.11 (−0.22)*	This result is within normal range for his age.
NIA conventional	0 (1)*	The mode for this score is 0 as most typically developing children do not imitate the examiner as they do not need a model to play.
NIA symbolic	1 (1)*	The mode for this score is 0 as most typically developing children do not imitate the examiner as they do not need a model to play. A score of 1 is still within normal range.
NIA combined	1 (2)*	The mode for this score is 0 as most typically developing children do not imitate the examiner as they do not need a model to play. A score of 1 is still within normal range of 0–2.

Key: *Scores from initial assessment (See Table 8.2); PEPA: percentage of elaborate pretend play actions; NOS: number of object substitutions; NIA: number of imitated actions; Conventional: the scores relate to the conventional imaginative play session of the ChIPPA; Symbolic: the scores relate to the symbolic play session of the ChIPPA; Combined: the scores relate to the conventional imaginative play session plus the symbolic play session of the ChIPPA

show where gardens are redesigned. In these play scenes he was the boss who organized the other workers!

8.4 Conclusion

Play is a child's primary occupation. A child's occupational performance in pretend play impacts on how a child interacts with others, understands others and how he or she prepares for literacy skills at school. Language and social competence are also reflected in the occupation of pretend play. A new approach to assessing the occupational performance of play has been developed where a child's ability to self-initiate pretend play can be determined by measuring the complexity of a child's play, the child's ability to use symbols in play, whether a child can initiate play, and observations relating to the quality of play such as time played and use of narrative. Using the ChIPPA as a single assessment or as part of a battery of assessments, assists the therapist and child's carers to identify occupational performance issues such as:

- A lack of ability in pretend play (due to either occupational performance components or occupational deprivation or both).
- Inability to pretend play due to circumstances such as lack of access to space to play, lack of play materials, attitudes of carers, cultural restrictions (occupational justice).
- Lack of play ability due to excess time spent in other occupations such as activities of daily living (occupational imbalance).
- Ability to play with only one type of play material such as cars (occupational alienation).

By identifying the issues in occupational performance of pretend play, the child's pretend play can then be enabled either by changes to environmental circumstances and/or use of the Learn to Play programme. The Learn to Play programme enables occupational performance in pretend play by providing developmental levels of play, suggested play materials and emphasis on the child's ability to self-initiate play ideas.

A case example was given of a child diagnosed with autism spectrum disorder to demonstrate the assessment of pretend play as a unique occupation and the value of occupational treatment by enabling a child to play. For children who have occupational performance issues in pretend play, enhancing their ability to play improves the child's quality of life and enables him or her to participate in society to a greater degree than previously.

References

Baron-Cohen, S. (1996). *Mindblindness. An Essay on Autism and Theory of Mind.* MIT Press: London.

Bledsoe, N. & Shepherd, J.T. (1982). A study of reliability and validity of a pre-school play scale. *American Journal of Occupational Therapy, 36,* 783–787.

Bracegirdle, H. (1992). The use of play in occupational therapy for children: what is play? *British Journal of Occupational Therapy, 55,* 107–108.

Bundy, A.C. (1991). Play theory and sensory integration. In: E.A. Morrison, A.G. Fisher & A.C. Bundy (Eds), *Sensory Integration. Theory and Practice* (pp. 46–68). Philadelphia: F.A. Davis Company.

Bundy, A.C. (1993). Assessment of play and leisure: delineation of the problem. *American Journal of Occupational Therapy, 47,* 217–222.

Bundy, A. (1997). Play and playfulness: what to look for. In: L.D. Parham & L.S. Fazio (Eds), *Play in Occupational Therapy for Children* (pp. 52–66). St Louis: Mosby.

Bundy, A. (2001). Measuring play performance. In: M. Law, D. Baum & W. Dunn (Eds), *Measuring Occupational Performance. Supporting Best Practice in Occupational Therapy* (pp. 89–102). Thorofare, NJ: Slack Incorporated.

Canadian Association of Occupational Therapists (1996). Practice paper: occupational therapy and children's play. *Canadian Journal of Occupational Therapy, 63*, 1–9.

Casby, M.W. (1992). Symbolic play: development and assessment considerations. *Infants and Young Children, 4*, 43–48.

Couch, K.J., Deitz, J.C. & Kanny, E.M. (1997). The role of play in paediatric occupational therapy. *American Journal of Occupational Therapy, 52*, 111–117.

Cross, L.A. & Coster, W.J. (1997). Symbolic play language during sensory integration treatment. *American Journal of Occupational Therapy, 51*, 808–814.

Fein, G.G. (1975). A transformational analysis of pretending. *Developmental Psychology, 11*, 291–296.

Goodman, J.F. (1994). 'Work' versus 'play' and early childhood care. *Early Childhood Care, 23*, 177–196.

Haight, W.L. & Miller, P.J. (1993). *Pretending at Home. Early Development in the Socio-cultural Context.* Albany: State University of New York Press.

Howard, A.C. (1986). Developmental play ages of physically abused and non-abused children. *American Journal of Occupational Therapy, 40*, 691–694.

Humphry, R. (2002). Young children's occupations: explicating the dynamics of developmental processes. *American Journal of Occupational Therapy, 56*, 171–179.

Knox, S.H. (1974). A play scale. In: M. Reilly (Ed.), *Play as Exploratory Learning: Studies of Curiosity Behaviour* (pp. 247–266). Beverley Hills: Sage Publications.

Lewis, V. & Boucher, J. (1997). *The Test of Pretend Play. Manual.* London: Psychological Services.

Lewis, V., Boucher, J. & Astell, A. (1992). The assessment of symbolic play in young children: a prototype test. *European Journal of Disorders of Communications, 27*, 231–245.

Lewis, V., Boucher, J., Lupton, L. & Watson, S. (2000). Notes and discussion. Relationships between symbolic play, functional play and symbolic play in young children. *International Journal of Language and Communication Disorders, 35*, 117–127.

McCune Nicolich, L. (1977). Beyond sensorimotor intelligence: assessment of symbolic maturity through analysis of pretend play. *Merrill-Palmer Quarterly, 23*, 89–99.

Michelman, S.S. (1974). Play and the deficit child. In: M. Reilly (Ed.), *Play as Exploratory Learning: Studies in Curiosity Behaviour* (pp. 157–207). Beverley Hills: Sage Publications.

Parham, L.D. & Primeau, L.A. (1997). Play and occupational therapy. In: L.D. Parham & L.S. Fazio (Eds), *Play in Occupational Therapy for Children* (pp. 2–21). St Louis: Mosby.

Pellegrini, A.D. & Galda, L. (1993). Ten years after: a re-examination of symbolic play and literacy research. *Reading Research Quarterly, 28*, 162–175.

Piaget, J. (1962). *Play, Dreams and Imitation in Childhood.* New York: W.W. Norton & Company.

Pierce, D. (1997). The power of object play for infants and toddlers at risk for developmental delay. In: L.D. Parham & L.S. Fazio (Eds), *Play in Occupational Therapy for Children* (pp. 86–111). St Louis: Mosby.

Power, T. & Radcliffe, J. (1991). Cognitive assessment of pre-school play using the symbolic play test. In: C. Schaefer, K. Gitlin & A. Sandgrund (Eds), *Play Diagnosis and Assessment* (pp. 87–111). New York: John Wiley & Sons Inc.

Reid, D. (1987). Occupational therapists' assessment practices with handicapped children in Ontario. *Canadian Journal of Occupational Therapy, 54,* 181–187.

Reilly, M. (1974a). *Play as Exploratory Learning. Studies in Curiosity Behaviour.* Beverley Hills: Sage Publishers.

Reilly, M. (1974b). An explanation of play. In: M. Reilly (Ed.), *Play as Exploratory Learning. Studies in Curiosity Behaviour* (pp. 117–155). Beverley Hills: Sage Publications.

de Renne-Stephan, C. (1980). Imitation: a mechanism of play behaviour. *American Journal of Occupational Therapy, 34,* 95–102.

Robinson, A.L. (1977). Play: the arena for acquisition of rules for competent behaviour. *American Journal of Occupational Therapy, 31,* 248–253.

Rodger, S. (1994). A survey of assessments used by paediatric occupational therapists. *Australian Occupational Therapy Journal, 41,* 137–142.

Rodger, S. & Ziviani, J. (1999). Play-based occupational therapy. *International Journal of Disability, Development and Education, 46,* 337–365.

Rubin, K., Fein, G. & Vandenberg, B. (1983). Play. In: P.H. Mussen (Series Ed.), *Handbook of Child Psychology: Socialization, Personality and Social Development* (4th edn) Vol. 4, pp. 693–774. New York: Wiley.

Schrader, C.T. (1989). Written language use within the context of young children's symbolic play. *Early Childhood Research Quarterly, 4,* 225–244.

Sherratt, D. (2002). Developing pretend play in children with autism. *SAGE Publications and the National Autistic Society, 6,* 169–179.

Sparling, J.W., Walker, D.F. & Singdahlsen, J. (1984). Play techniques with neurologically impaired pre-schoolers. *American Journal of Occupational Therapy, 38,* 603–612.

Stagnitti, K. (1998). *Learn to Play. A Practical Programme to Develop a Child's Imaginative Play Skills.* Melbourne: Coordinates Publications.

Stagnitti, K. (2002). The development of a child-initiated assessment of pretend play. Vol. 1. Unpublished PhD thesis, La Trobe University, Melbourne, Australia.

Stagnitti, K. & Unsworth, C. (2000). The importance of pretend play in child development. *British Journal of Occupational Therapy, 63,* 121–127.

Stagnitti, K., Unsworth, C. & Rodger, S. (2000). Development of an assessment to identify play behaviours that discriminate between the play of typical preschoolers and pre-schoolers with pre-academic problems. *Canadian Journal of Occupational Therapy, 67,* 291–303.

Stewart, D., Harvey, S., Sahagian, S., Toal, C., Pollock, N. & Law, M. (1991). *Play: the Occupation of Childhood.* Hamilton, Ontario; Neurodevelopmental Clinical Research Unit, The Ontario Ministry of Health.

Ungerer, J.A., Zelazo, P.R., Kearsley, R.B. & O'Leary, K. (1981). Developmental changes in the representation of objects in symbolic play from 18 to 34 months of age. *Child Development, 52,* 186–195.

Vandenberg, B. & Kielhofner, G. (1982). Play in evolution, culture and individual adaptation: implications for therapy. *American Journal of Occupational Therapy, 36,* 20–28.

VORT Corporation (1995). *HELP for Pre-schoolers. Assessment & Curriculum Guide.* Palo Alto: VORT Corporation.

Vygotsky, L.S. (1966). Play and its role in the mental development of the child. *Voprosy psikhologii* (Soviet Psychology), *12,* 62–76.

Vygotsky, L. (1997). *Thought and Language* (A. Kozulin, Trans.). Mass.: the MIT Press.

Westby, C. (1991). A scale for assessing children's pretend play. In: C. Schaefer, K. Gitlin & A. Sandgrund (Eds), *Play Diagnosis and Assessment* (pp. 131–161). New York: John Wiley & Sons Inc.

World Health Organization. (2001). *International Classification of Functioning*. Geneva: WHO.

Wyver, S. & Spence, S. (1995). Cognitive and social play of Australian pre-schoolers. *Australian Journal of Early Childhood*, 20, 42–46.

von Zuben, M.V., Crist, P.A. & Mayberry, W. (1991). A pilot study of differences in play behaviour between children of low and middle socio-economic status. *American Journal of Occupational Therapy*, 45, 113–119.

Chapter 9

Social Inclusion through Occupation in Community Mental Health

Rachel Hayden

9.1 Introduction

This chapter provides in detail an example of practice carried out within a community mental health setting and demonstrates how occupational therapy theory and occupational science can provide the rationale and the evidence to support occupational therapy in practice. Treatment within a group setting is a frequent approach used by mental health occupational therapists. This chapter outlines an example of community-based group work in practice and focuses on the assessment and experiences of two particular individuals. These individuals, although unique in themselves, had similar needs that the group aimed to address. The Occupational Performance History Interview, version II (OPHI-II) (Kielhofner *et al.*, 1998), was used as the assessment tool to identify individuals' occupational strengths, needs and volitional narratives prior to their referral to the group. The Model of Human Occupation, a framework which maintains a focus on occupation and which is supported by occupational theory and research, underpins this assessment tool (Kielhofner, 1995). The functional group model (Howe & Schwarzberg, 2001), based on research and theoretical assumptions from group dynamics and occupational therapy, provided a framework for the design and process of the group.

9.2 Overview of practice context

Occupational therapy evolved from the field of mental health, but much has changed since those early days. The environments in which mental health occupational therapists work are very different, but the assumptions which underpin practice remain the same and are being re-harnessed and re-energised. Changes in health and social care in the UK have meant that most people with mental health problems are being supported in the community. Service providers are listening to service users and attempting to meet their self-identified needs

(Department of Health, 1990, 1999). These needs include, but are not limited to, engaging in society, enjoying mainstream leisure, education and work opportunities, and access to community facilities (Department of Health, 1999). The transition from institutionalized, service-led provision to community-based user-led care is a welcome shift in philosophy for occupational therapists, who hold the principle of client-centred intervention at the core of their profession (Canadian Association of Occupational Therapists, 1991; Sumsion, 1999; College of Occupational Therapists, 2000).

Despite the demand from service users and service providers for interventions that focus on occupational engagement and social inclusion, occupational therapists in community mental health settings continue to struggle in defining their role and maintaining an occupational focus in practice. Meeson's study (1998a) of twelve occupational therapists within community mental health teams (CMHTs) in the UK found that they favoured interventions such as supported counselling, anxiety management and problem solving rather than occupationally focused interventions. Despite being a small study, it reflected the concerns of the profession regarding role blurring and a greater emphasis on generic working within these environments (Craik *et al.*, 1998; Taylor & Rubin, 1999; Hughes, 2001; Parker, 2001). In fact, the College of Occupational Therapists found it necessary to state that 'Occupational therapists should spend the majority of their clinical time working as occupational therapists and not as generalist mental health workers' (Craik *et al.*, 1998, p. 391). Numerous suggestions have been made as to why occupational therapists struggle to adhere to their specialist role. These include role ambiguity, role conflict, role blurring and an inability of occupational therapists to defend their specialist contribution (Feaver & Creek, 1993; Kwai-sang Yau, 1995; Meeson, 1998b; Craik *et al.*, 1999; Hughes, 2001; Molineux, 2002a).

The National Service Framework for Mental Health (Department of Health, 1999), a Government document outlining the structure of and requirements for the development of mental health care provision in the UK, has provided a clarity of purpose for many mental health teams. New primary care based mental health care teams are emerging, to meet the demands from general practitioners for services for their many patients with common mental health problems, such as anxiety and depression. The establishment of these teams allows CMHTs to focus on the needs of people with severe and enduring mental health difficulties (Department of Health, 1999). The Sainsbury Centre for Mental Health (2001) report, commissioned to complement the National Service Framework, identifies the capabilities that all mental health practitioners should possess. It also outlines 'best practice' specialist mental health interventions but does not specify which profession's remit these fall under. However, the social and practical interventions outlined in the document fit well with occupational therapy philosophy and approaches. The capabilities in this section are (Sainsbury Centre for Mental Health, 2001, p. 17):

- Identifying and collaborating with the range of local specialist and non-specialist community resources available to service users and their families to assist them to maintain quality of life (including work, education and leisure).

- Creating, developing and maintaining the personal and social networks of service users and their carers and families.
- Providing advice, assistance or training in daily living skills, for clients and their carers and families.

In this context, occupational therapists in the UK have a valuable opportunity to demonstrate their worth to clients with mental health difficulties living in the community. Occupational science provides occupational therapists with knowledge to support their practice in the field. Occupational therapists must demonstrate their knowledge and use of occupation in their practice, highlight their specialist skills and illustrate how their unique focus can meet the needs of service users. If they fail to do this, other disciplines may develop these roles for themselves (Morgan, 1993; Molineux, 2002b).

9.3   Establishing client need

Like others, individuals with severe and enduring mental health problems desire to feel a sense of belonging, acceptance, autonomy, being valued and being productive (Grady, 1995; Laliberte-Rudman *et al.*, 2000; Rebeiro *et al.*, 2000). However, for people with a diagnosis of schizophrenia, for example, these needs frequently remain unmet (Strathdee *et al.*, 1997; Laliberte-Rudman *et al.*, 2000; Rebeiro *et al.*, 2000). Not only disabled by their symptoms, or by the side effects of medication, such individuals are outcasts in a world that does not tolerate difference (Grady, 1995). These individuals, who live in a community that is ill-equipped to accommodate them, need to feel the very real inclusion that service providers talk about but frequently struggle to deliver (Dunn, 1999; Wright, 2000; Wright & De Ponte, 2000; Payne, 2002).

The needs of Pushpa and Simon, who were both referred to the occupational therapist by their community psychiatric nurse (CPN), were no different. Pushpa was referred to the community resources group, which was being set up jointly by the occupational therapist and a CPN. She wanted to develop her skills in accessing community facilities so that she could widen her leisure and social activities. Simon was initially referred to the occupational therapist for an assessment of his skills with a view to possible future employment.

Whilst checklists for roles and interests, and daily activity records indicate areas of need and a baseline for re-evaluation, drawing on clients' personal narratives is being encouraged (Clark, 1993; Helfrich *et al.*, 1994). The art of identifying clients' needs involves an in-depth understanding of each individual's perception of themselves as an occupational being, and of the disparity that may exist between their present sense of self and what they once were, or what they hoped to become. The most effective way of establishing this disparity is for the therapist and client to return to a time when the client identified himself/herself as balanced, growing and able to engage in affirming occupations. This occupational storytelling will highlight for the client and the therapist the richness and wholeness once evident in the person, and the significant losses that they have encountered through their journey of mental ill health (Clark, 1993; Helfrich *et al.*, 1994; Mattingly, 1998). Clark (1993, p. 1074) tells us that 'occupational storytelling is a means by which therapists better understand the spirit of the survivors with whom they work'. Using the Occupational Performance History Interview, version II (Kielhofner, *et al.*, 1998) the occupational therapist was able to contextualize the occupational performance needs of Pushpa and Simon in their environments and their life narratives.

9.3.1   Pushpa's story

Pushpa, a 32 year-old British Asian woman, was diagnosed with schizophrenia when she was 21. The oldest of four daughters, she was the only one still living with her parents. Her youngest sister was studying at university, her middle sister was a holiday representative and her eldest sister was married with her own children. Pushpa wanted to be a laboratory technician, but since her first acute psychotic episode whilst at college studying for her GCSEs at the age of 18, she had been unable to move towards realizing her dream. A typical day for Pushpa involved rising mid-morning, eating breakfast, carrying out a few chores, helping with lunch, watching television, eating dinner and going to bed at 10.00 pm. The only variety in Pushpa's timetable occurred when there were different self-care or home maintenance tasks to perform, such as running errands for her mother or changing her bed linen.

Pushpa's positive symptoms were controlled by medication, in that she rarely heard voices or had delusional beliefs. Her motivation was reduced, she fatigued easily, lacked confidence in her abilities and was experiencing symp-toms of anxiety. Pushpa was frightened to engage in activities outside her home or familiar mental health settings and often remained at home with her mother who did not like to be left alone. Pushpa would not use public transport or go into town unless accompanied. When her sisters were home Pushpa seemed to come alive, she would go shopping for clothes, help prepare for family parties, and go tenpin bowling or to the movies. As they grew older, however, Pushpa and her sisters began moving in different directions, and did not see each other as frequently.

Pushpa had numerous goals and interests. She wanted a professional job, a partner and family, and her own home. She was, however, stuck in a chapter of her life in which she only ever danced with these aspirations. She started many courses, only to drop out, she felt too afraid to move out of her parents' house, and her identity was dependent on the varying expectations of those around her. Adulthood is characterized by the development of a sense of personal identity, the ability to engage in a truly intimate relationship, and engagement in productive occupations (Erikson, 1980; Kielhofner, 1995). As schizophrenia tends to have an onset in late adolescence (Jablensky, 2000) it can have a profound effect on one's ability to move into this next phase of development. Pushpa was intelligent, ambitious, sociable and creative, but struggled to move into adulthood.

9.3.2   Simon's story

Simon graduated in 1984 with a Bachelor's degree in fine art, at the age of 21. It was some three years after this that he had his first psychotic episode and was later diagnosed as having schizophrenia. On passing his degree, and not being accepted onto a postgraduate course, he felt he lost his direction and worked in a burger bar. Simon worked in various jobs for the first few years of his illness, whilst living with his parents. The work in factories, food outlets and bars was casual and poorly paid, with limited prospects. This was in contrast to Simon's siblings, who were both successful in their careers and married with families of their own. Simon wanted these things for himself, but felt that he would never be able to attain them.

In 1993, after only brief periods in hospital, Simon's mental state deteriorated considerably. He heard voices, believed he was poisoning others and that the FBI were after him. He cut his wrists and jumped through a window, sustaining a fractured skull. Following a period of time in medical intensive care he was discharged to a psychiatric hospital and from there to a hostel. Simon had his own combined bedroom/living room and kitchen, but shared the bathroom and laundry facilities. His daily routine became similar to Pushpa's, in that most of his occupations related to self-care and home maintenance.

Simon had acquired additional qualifications in music, word processing, desktop publishing and media studies since the first onset of his illness. When asked to identify his skills, however, he cited cooking, shopping, cashing in his benefit book and taking his medication at the right time each day. Simon described getting a job and having a girlfriend as 'just a dream', and when asked what he saw himself doing in five to ten years time he said 'Do you make your own destiny? ... I let things happen to me ... I let things wash over me.' The motivation for occupational engagement is influenced by our belief that we can be successful and master the challenges that we face (Keilhofner, 1995). Simon no longer felt like the author of his volitional narrative, he had a limited sense of self-efficacy, did not feel in control of his life and this affected the occupational choices that he made. Simon identified himself with the mundane tasks of his daily life and thus cited the skills he had in relation to these. His previous abilities and achievements were not congruent with his current sense of self as an occupational being.

Having not transitioned fully into adulthood, Simon and Pushpa remained refugees displaced from their life course (Bateson, 1990) by the impact of their illness. Simon and Pushpa (with help from her family) were able to manage their daily living occupations and sustain themselves in the community. Nonetheless, their quality of life, sense of belonging and their opportunity to engage in social occupations were severely restricted. Social occupations require a social network, and the environments in which we live can impede or facilitate our occupational performance (Grady, 1995; Kielhofner, 1995; Gray, 1998; Wilcock, 1998; Wood, 2002). The OPHI-II assessment highlights the impact of context on occupational identity and competence using the Occupational Behaviour Settings Scale.

Pushpa's occupational behaviour setting improved dramatically when her sisters were at home, allowing her to utilize her skills and pursue her interests. Simon maintained very limited behaviour settings and was cautious about engaging in social occupations. As a consequence he became even less skilled and confident in his abilities. Neither individual had a social network outside their families that would give them a wider sense of community and a place to express their true occupational selves.

Passmore's (1998) study identified that participation in social leisure activities, chosen freely by the participant and challenging in nature, helped to develop skills relating to relationships and social acceptance. She also found that this positively influenced self-esteem and prepared individuals for future worker roles. It is no surprise, therefore, that without meaningful productivity or leisure occupations Pushpa and Simon's occupational identity and competence would be affected. The OPHI-II assessment revealed occupational dysfunction in both these areas for both individuals. Pushpa wanted to work but lacked commitment to any future goals or projects, unclear about what she was capable of and what was expected of her. Simon valued the status of employment but had limited expectations of success in his ability to fulfil a worker role, and therefore disregarded this as a realistic option. The courses that he had successfully completed since his illness had not assisted him in broadening his social community and he remained shy and introverted, struggling with social relationships. Pushpa had some confidence in mixing with others but struggled to motivate herself and access social environments outside her family circle and so both individuals identified a need to develop their roles as friends and participants in the wider community.

Although there were many occupational deficits identified in Pushpa and Simon's narratives, addressing their social needs was a primary goal that had meaning for both of them. The occupational therapist proposed that they could use the community resources group to assist them in meeting these needs. Wilcock (1998, p. 104) states that: 'Social well-being will be enhanced if people are able to develop their potential through practice in a range of socially valued occupations.' The community resource group provided a new occupational behaviour setting for Pushpa and Simon.

9.4   Intervention planning

In the study by Laliberte-Rudman *et al.* (2000) of quality of life of people with schizophrenia, informants identified that part of the theme of connecting and belonging involved being perceived as normal. This included being part of a community and being involved in social activities that were typical for the general population. The importance of ensuring that intervention is provided in a real context is not to be underestimated (Gray, 1998). The community resources group aimed to provide an opportunity for group members to gain a sense of belonging, develop friendships, exercise choice and participate in normal social occupations within their community. These included, for example, tenpin bowling, boating, and visits to local parks and places of interest. The group did not use health service transport or present themselves to any of the community facilities as a group with special needs.

9.4.1   The group process

The aims of the group were addressed by utilizing occupation and the group process to effect change. Specifically, the functional group model, which draws on occupational therapy and group dynamics (Howe & Schwartzberg, 2001), provided a framework for the group. The model aims to enhance the occupational behaviour of group participants through shared, client-centred occupation. Attention is paid to the group environment and how the roles and responsibilities within the group impact on group cohesion and performance. Members need to learn to be aware of their own and each other's strengths and needs. This involves the development of self-awareness and effective communication skills. Group facilitators need to be aware of this process and to recognize that their style of facilitation could influence the overall performance of the group.

The functional group model proposes that the group leader is initially responsible for planning, and as the group members develop their skills and responsibilities the leader gradually hands the responsibility of decision making over to its members. In the community resources group, the members met for a number of planning sessions. The facilitators devised a loose structure for these sessions, anticipating that the structure would evolve as the group members became more confident and comfortable with the process. Warm-up activities were planned to begin each session, aimed at relaxing participants and promoting interaction and cohesion. The session aims and plan were presented at the start of the group, and each participant had an opportunity to clarify or add to the aims. At the end of the session an agenda was devised for the following week and participants were asked to share thoughts or comments on the session.

Howe and Schwartzberg (2001) cite Robert White's (1959) examination of 'effectance motivation' as central to the development of the functional group model. White suggested that exploratory behaviour was self-motivated and had adaptive value. The model predicts that the structure of functional groups will motivate members to purposeful and meaningful action. The occupation taking place in the planning stage of the group was less active but no less meaningful, as members developed and implemented skills in socializing, decision making, problem solving, goal setting, evaluating and reflecting. In many respects these planning sessions enhanced the occupational performance components required for the activity that followed. These sessions provided a safe and supportive environment in which participants could explore all the elements required for successful engagement in a community outing. It was envisaged that after three planning sessions the group would be prepared to engage in an occupation in the community. Every fourth week, therefore, the group format changed depending on the occupation that had been chosen, and members would enjoy participating in the end product. Howe and Schwartzberg's (2001) model proposes that functional groups do not only exist in a therapeutic setting but apply to naturally occurring groups in the community. One aim of the community resources group was, therefore, to facilitate an environment that mirrored that of natural groups.

The overall aims of the group were outlined to Pushpa and Simon following assessment and they both recognized that the group might assist them in meeting their needs. More specific individual objectives were identified within the group sessions. This approach aimed to assist in the development of group cohesiveness and allowed individuals to share their difficulties and support each other in achieving their personal objectives. The Binary Individualized Outcome Measure (Cook & Spreadbury, 1995) was used within the sessions to assist in this process. This measure was chosen because it is client-centred and simple to use, in that participants can take an active role in identifying and monitoring their achievements.

9.5   Implementing the intervention

The group began with six members, all of whom were assessed by the occupational therapist and the CPN. The optimal size of the group is an important consideration and depends on the kind of work being carried out. Finlay (1993) recommends eight or more members for a social group and four to six for a task group. A core membership of six, however, was maintained throughout most of the group's 18-month history. The needs of other individuals assessed for the group were broadly similar to those of Pushpa and Simon, that is, they were relatively stable in their mental state but constraints in their occupational behaviour settings provided them with little opportunity to engage effectively in meaningful social occupations.

In the first few weekly sessions, facilitators took on most of the responsibilities, structuring the session and leading the group exercises. In the initial sessions group members introduced themselves to each other and talked about their interests and what they felt constituted a community. The main focus of the group was about accessing community resources. It was important that the group members, not the facilitators, outlined what that term meant to them. This handing over of responsibility assisted in establishing the client-centred ethos of the group (Sumsion, 1999). On establishing that the library was a useful resource for obtaining information, a library visit became the first planned outing. The local library was already known to some participants and so, with an emphasis on skill sharing and mutual support, some group members agreed to rendezvous at a particular location and go to the library together. Other less confident members chose to meet at the neighbourhood centre and travel with the facilitators. Having group members with similar needs but mixed abilities evoked a sense of shared responsibility. Simon, for example, was initially very quiet in the group, but was confident to meet up with another group member for this exercise. On the other hand, Pushpa, who was more sociable in the group, initially preferred to be supported by group facilitators.

As the planning sessions continued, ground rules were established in order to clarify expectations of behaviour within the group. Facilitators stressed, for example, that the choice of occupation would need to be made by the group as a whole. It was agreed that this would be done democratically with a range of ideas being put to the vote. Initially the facilitators voted for occupations as well, and by doing so were able to demonstrate that a difference of opinion was acceptable. Another ground rule was that all occupations needed to be ultimately achievable without financial or practical assistance from the facilitators. This was important if the occupations carried out were to be sustainable independently from the facilitators. Most of the group members did not drive and all were on benefits, and so developing skills in using public transport and budgeting were important goals of the group. A behavioural norm, which developed spontaneously, was that people rarely discussed their illness. The group members perceived the sessions to be fun, positive and normalizing, and an opportunity for them to engage in something that wasn't about their illness. The group developed a very relaxed and sociable atmosphere; this was helped by the warm-up exercises, which became a regular feature in the group meetings. Members gradually took on the role of devising warm-up exercises each week, asking questions such as, 'If you could meet anyone in the world alive or dead who would it be?' or, 'If you won the lottery what would you spend your money on?' These activities reinforced members' self-identities as individuals and their occupational natures began to emerge and were embraced.

Individual skills also came to light during the planning sessions. Pushpa, who was discovered to be good at maths, took on the role of treasurer and collected money for tea and coffee. She also became quite a skilled minute taker, a role that developed as the group realized that they were forgetting some of the ideas being discussed. Simon was thorough in gathering information and could be relied upon to bring detailed resource information for discussion. He also used his art skills when asked by other members to design a group logo. Simon took this role seriously and presented the group with a portfolio of ideas from which they could choose. One logo was chosen and was used in all future group posters, evaluation forms and other paperwork used by the group.

The only roles that Pushpa and Simon identified prior to attending the group were that of home maintainer and family member. These roles limited their occupational performance and provided them with few challenges to develop their occupational lifestyles. The group roles they assumed, although small, allowed them to express themselves and use their talents. For Simon they also influenced what he did outside the group and pressed his normal routine as he prepared ideas for the next group session. Pushpa tended to avoid preparatory work outside the session, but embraced her roles within the immediacy of the group meetings. However, on the occasions when group members brought in food to share, Pushpa rose to the challenge and prepared samosas, bhajis and home-made Bombay mix. This occupational form (Kielhofner & Barrett, 1997) held meaning and value for her and provided her with the opportunity to share her culture with others, reinforcing her cultural identity. It also reinforced a positive role identity for her as a daughter, as Pushpa and her mother often worked together on providing refreshments for the group. These positive definitions of herself influenced Pushpa's occupational identity by enabling her to enact a role that focused on her own strengths.

Initially, occupations chosen by the group were familiar to participants, such as going for a walk at a local beauty spot and going to the cinema. As roles, routines and habits developed, members became more comfortable and ideas brought to the group for discussion gradually became more challenging. Grady (1995) conceptualizes this progression as a spiralling continuum in which a person travels from dependence to interdependence. The spiral begins with a holding environment, a safe place where individuals experience a strong sense of attachment and belonging. Individuals then move into a facilitating environment that aims to provide just enough support to move into new situations. With successful adaptation, members of the group moved into a challenging environment where they could test their potential. Grady (1995, p. 306) states that 'just the right amount of challenge is needed if the person is to make an adaptive response to the situation'. The spiral peaks in an interactive environment where individuals are able to develop self-awareness and recognize the benefits of relationships with others. Recognition of this process and identification of where group members placed themselves on this spiral assisted with the ongoing evaluation of the group.

The group continued for 18 months in total, with reviews every 12 weeks. During that time the group visited country parks, bird sanctuaries, art galleries and gardens, and went on to horse riding, quad biking, boating and go-kart racing. Each occupation elicited and reinforced skills, interests and challenges for different group members. The facilitators encouraged participants to carry on these occupations with each other or with other family members or friends outside the group setting. Pushpa enjoyed the go-karting so much that she arranged the activity with her sisters when they returned home one weekend. Following the onset of her illness, Pushpa had identified frustration at her perceived loss of status as the eldest sister. Leading her sisters in go-karting, which was new to them but familiar to her, provided Pushpa with the opportunity to make a link with her past occupational identity.

As the group progressed and members' skills and confidence developed, the facilitators gradually withdrew. Participants took turns in facilitating the group, and rather than travelling to an activity as a whole group, members met at bus stops or train stations, and met the facilitators at the destination. As time went on, the facilitators withdrew from the outings altogether, and were eager to hear about them at the next group meeting. As outings became easier to plan, the group no longer required three weeks to organize themselves, and so they used the sessions to support each other in the pursuit of their personal objectives. Simon, for example, wanted to improve his fitness, and set an objective to join the local leisure centre and go swimming once a week. Group members supported Simon by providing him with information on swimming pools in his local area, and suggesting ways he could save money by getting a leisure card. One member, who had been to the local pool before, agreed to go with him on the first few occasions until he felt confident with the routine.

9.6   Evaluation and discharge

Wilcock (1993, p. 18) states that 'occupation provides the mechanism for social interaction, and social development and growth, forming the foundation stone of communal, local and national identity'. The community resources group provided an environment whereby Pushpa and Simon were able to explore and develop their social occupations and enhance their occupational identities and competence. In their final evaluation statements both remarked that through the group they felt they had gained friends and confidence. Simon stated: 'I feel more at ease with myself and with others generally, and am therefore happier with myself.' This suggests that, in the context of the group, Simon had been able to experience Grady's interactive environment (1995). He maintained friendships with some of the group members long after the facilitators had withdrawn, and these continue. Although Pushpa also acknowledged that she had gained friends from the group, she required external motivation. In her evaluation she highlighted the skills she had gained from attending the group: 'Planning activities, finding out about things like the buses and alternative transport in getting somewhere I would really like to go.' Whereas 'before, I just wouldn't do it'. The attainment of these skills increased her confidence, but Pushpa had not attained what Grady (1995, p. 306) called 'interdependence'. She would not maintain engagement in activities outside her home without encouragement. Pushpa's overall attendance at the group had been sporadic and she was skilled in providing reasons either for her non-attendance or for not achieving goals she had set for herself. While Pushpa did not achieve sustained social interactions and community independence outside the group, she did gain a great deal from her here-and-now experiences.

In evaluating the group, the facilitators revisited their original aims and felt that these had been achieved. Most of the group members no longer required support from the facilitators to access and engage in community based leisure occupations. Participants in the group reviews reinforced this opinion when verbal feedback was obtained. Individual objectives, identified by the Binary Individualized Outcome Measure (Cook & Spreadbury, 1995), demonstrated that the majority of regular participants had achieved most of the goals they had set for themselves and were continuing to set future goals independently. Pushpa and Simon engaged in occupations that were challenging to them, and acknowledged the progress they had made and the confidence they had gained. By successfully mastering these challenges Pushpa and Simon identified improvements in their self-esteem and for Simon in particular, this increased his belief in his skills and altered his outlook regarding his future. The experience of the group widened their community, allowing them to be connected to others.

The group disbanded with a farewell lunch at a local pub. No lengthy planning was required, and all members made their way to the venue without facilitator support. Many members had now become involved in other occupations and were already planning their next outing as a group. They agreed to meet in four weeks time in the town centre and go tenpin bowling. When one of the facilitators met with an ex-group member some months later, she was told that a few of them still met periodically, and Simon continued to see one friend he had made in the group, on a weekly basis. Simon still felt unable to consider employment but had joined an art class at a local neighbourhood centre. Pushpa continued to receive occupational therapy input on a one-to-one basis, as she wanted to develop her independent living skills, particularly in relation to cooking and shopping. She also attended a sheltered mental health education project, participating in a volunteer training course although her attendance continued to be sporadic. Following the death of her father, Pushpa moved with her mother to another side of town, within a supportive Asian community, and was no longer dancing with, but living her aspirations, as she was regularly attending mainstream college.

9.7   Conclusion

Meeting the needs of individuals with severe and enduring mental health problems can be challenging. Humans are complex, unpredictable and unique, and mental health service users are no different. Humans also, however, like things to be straightforward, predictable and often struggle with change. It is perhaps understandable, therefore, that professionals, including occupational therapists, seek to engage in work with service users that is structured, easy to achieve and simple to measure. Perhaps that is why so many occupational therapists stick to anxiety management, and similarly regimented interventions. Occupation is often perceived as mundane because it is commonplace and usually taken for granted. Occupation is a complex phenomenon and occupational therapists have fallen into the trap of breaking it down into component parts and addressing dysfunction as merely a collection of skill deficits.

This chapter has demonstrated how occupational therapists can begin to acknowledge the complex occupational needs of clients with mental health difficulties and start to address the social exclusion that comes with severe and enduring mental illness, through the use of occupation. Occupational science and occupational therapy theory provide the guiding light that can steer the therapist through these complexities. Mattingly's (1998) exploration in the use of narrative provides us with a mechanism by which we can encapsulate the richness of someone's life story that no checklist of functional abilities can come close to. The OPHI-II assessment enables therapists to draw on this occupational narrative and gain a better understanding of how occupational performance can be influenced by the values and meanings attributed to past events and environmental context. The intervention choice for Pushpa and Simon reflected these findings and the community resources group created an environment in which occupational engagement could be experienced in a context that was meaningful and sustainable after therapy.

At the end of the intervention Pushpa and Simon still experienced some degree of social exclusion, and neither were free from their dependency on mental health services. However, the community resources group enabled them to experience normal, enjoyable and challenging occupations that brought with them a sense of belonging and friendship. Research in occupational science demonstrates how these simple everyday experiences should not be underestimated but make up the essential elements that sustain well-being. It is this understanding that occupational therapists must promote within their working environments.

As occupational therapists we have the knowledge base and the skills to make a significant contribution to mental health services that are struggling to address the problem of social exclusion. With this wealth of knowledge at our fingertips, and with a brave step away from the old ways of working and into the new, we can maintain occupation at the heart of our interventions for the benefit of mental health service users.

References

Bateson, M. (1990). *Composing a Life*. New York: Plume.

Canadian Association of Occupational Therapists (1991). *Occupational Therapy Guidelines for Client-centred Practice*. Toronto: Canadian Association of Occupational Therapists.

Clark, F. (1993). Occupation embedded in a real life: interweaving occupational science and occupational therapy. *American Journal of Occupational Therapy, 47* (12), 1067–1078.

College of Occupational Therapists (2000). *Code of Ethics and Professional Conduct for Occupational Therapists*. London: College of Occupational Therapists.

Cook, S. & Spreadbury, P. (1995). *Measuring the Outcomes of Individualized Care: the Binary Individualized Outcome Measure*. Nottingham: Nottingham City Hospital NHS Trust.

Craik, C., Austin, C., Chacksfield, J., Richards, G. & Schell, D. (1998). College of Occupational Therapists position paper on the way ahead for research, education and practice in mental health. *British Journal of Occupational Therapy, 61* (9), 390–392.

Craik, C., Austin, C. & Schell, D. (1999). A national survey of occupational therapy managers in mental health. *British Journal of Occupational Therapy, 62* (5), 220–228.

Department of Health (1990). *NHS and Community Care Act 1990*. London: HMSO.

Department of Health (1999). *National Services Framework for Mental Health*. London: HMSO.

Dunn, S. (1999). *Creating Accepting Communities: Report of the Mind Inquiry into Social Exclusion*. London: Mind.

Erikson, E. (1980). *Identity and the Life Cycle*. New York: Norton.

Feaver, S. & Creek, J. (1993). Models of practice in occupational therapy: Part 2: what use are they? *British Journal of Occupational Therapy, 56* (2), 59–62.

Finlay, L. (1993). *Groupwork in Occupational Therapy*. Cheltenham: Nelson Thornes.

Grady, A. (1995). Building inclusive community: a challenge for occupational therapy. *American Journal of Occupational Therapy, 49* (4), 300–310.

Gray, J.M. (1998). Putting occupation into practice: occupation as ends, occupation as means. *American Journal of Occupational Therapy, 52* (5), 354–364.

Helfrich, C., Kielhofner, G. & Mattingly, C. (1994). Volition as narrative: Understanding motivation in chronic illness. *American Journal of Occupational Therapy, 48* (4), 311–317.

Howe, M.C. & Schwartzberg, S. (2001). *A Functional Approach to Group Work*, 3rd edn. Md.: Lippincott, Willliams & Wilkins.

Hughes, J. (2001). Occupational therapy in community mental health teams: a continuing dilemma? Role theory offers an explanation. *British Journal of Occupational Therapy, 64* (1), 34–40.

Jablensky, A. (2000) Epidemiology of schizophrenia. In: M. Gelder, J. Lopez-Ibor Jr, & N. Andreasen (Eds), *New Oxford Textbook of Psychiatry* (pp. 585–599). Oxford: Oxford University Press.

Kielhofner, G. (1995). *A Model of Human Occupation – Theory and Application*, 2nd edn. Baltimore: Williams & Wilkins.

Keilhofner, G. & Barrett, L. (1997). Meaning and misunderstanding in occupational forms: A study of therapeutic goal setting. *American Journal of Occupational Therapy, 52* (5), 345–353.

Kielhofner, G., Mallison, T., Crawford, C., Nowak, M., Rigby, M., Henry, A. & Walens, D. (1998). *A User's Manual for the Occupational Performance History Interview*. Chicago: The Model of Human Occupation Clearing House.

Kwai-sang Yau, M. (1995). Occupational therapy in community mental health: do we have a unique role in the interdisciplinary environment? *Australian Occupational Therapy Journal, 42*, 129–132.

Laliberte-Rudman, D., Yu, B., Scott, E. & Pajouhandeh, P. (2000). Exploration of the perspectives of persons with schizophrenia regarding quality of life. *American Journal of Occupational Therapy, 54* (2), 137–147.

Mattingly, C. (1998). *Healing Dramas and Clinical Plots – the Narrative Structure of Experience*. Cambridge: Cambridge University Press.

Meeson, B. (1998a). Occupational therapy in community mental health, Part 1: intervention choice. *British Journal of Occupational Therapy, 61* (1), 7–12.

Meeson, B. (1998b). Occupational therapy in community mental health, Part 2: factors influencing intervention choice. *British Journal of Occupational Therapy, 61* (2), 57–62.

Molineux, M. (2002a). Occupation and Occupational Therapy: Sorting out Some Issues. Keynote paper presented at the Annual Conference of the Association of Occupational Therapists in Mental Health, Leicester, UK.

Molineux, M. (2002b). The age of occupation: an opportunity to be seized. *MentalHealth OT, 7* (1), 12–14.

Morgan, S. (1993). *Community Mental Health – Practical Approaches to Long-term Problems*. London: Chapman and Hall.

Parker, H. (2001). The role of occupational therapists in community mental health teams: generic or specialist? *British Journal of Occupational Therapy, 64* (12), 609–611.

Passmore, A. (1998). Does leisure support and underpin adolescents' developing worker role? *Journal of Occupational Science, 5* (3), 161–165.

Payne, S. (2002). *Poverty, Social Exclusion and Mental Health: Findings from the 1999 Poverty and Social Exclusion Survey*. Bristol: Townsend Centre for International Poverty Research.

Rebeiro, K., Day, D., Semeniuk, B., O'Brien, M. & Wilson, B. (2000). Northern initiative for social action: an occupation-based mental health programme. *American Journal of Occupational Therapy, 55* (5), 493–500.

Sainsbury Centre for Mental Health (2001). *The Capable Practitioner Report*. London: Sainsbury Centre for Mental Health.

Strathdee, D., Thompson, K. & Carr, S. (1997). What service users want from mental health services. In: K. Thompson, D. Strathdee & D. Woods (Eds), *Mental Health Service Development Skills Workbook*. London: Sainsbury Centre for Mental Health.

Sumsion, T. (1999). Overview of client-centred practice. In T. Sumsion (Ed.), *Client-centred Practice in Occupational Therapy – a Guide to Implementation*. (pp. 1–14). Edinburgh: Churchill Livingstone.

Taylor, A. & Rubin, R. (1999). How do occupational therapists define their role in a community mental health setting? *British Journal of Occupational Therapy, 62* (2), 59–63.

Wilcock, A. (1993). A theory of the human need for occupation. *Journal of Occupational Science: Australia, 1* (1), 17–24.

Wilcock, A. (1998). *An Occupational Perspective of Health*. Thorofare: Slack.

Wood, W. (2002). Ecological synergies in two groups of zoo chimpanzees: divergent patterns of time use. *American Journal of Occupational Therapy, 56* (2), 160–170.

Wright, S. (2000). *'Is Anybody There?' A Survey of Friendship in Mental Health*. London: The Mental Health Foundation.

Wright, S. & De Ponte, P. (2000). *Pull Yourself Together! A Survey of the Stigma and Discrimination Faced by People who Experience Mental Distress*. London: The Mental Health Foundation.

Chapter 10
Occupational Reconstruction for People Living with HIV and AIDS

Sarah Yallop

10.1   Introduction

Occupational therapists have an important role to play in the services offered to care for people living with human immunodeficiency virus (HIV) and acquired immune deficiency syndrome (AIDS). Recent changes in monitoring and treatment have impacted on people living with HIV and AIDS and also those involved in providing health care. This chapter outlines the recent changes in the HIV context and the occupational impact of these changes using the example of Positive Employment Service, an occupational therapy service designed to address the reconstruction of productivity occupations for people living with HIV and AIDS. The focus of the chapter is on productivity occupations, but the issues discussed are also relevant for other occupations.

10.2   Overview: the changing context of HIV and AIDS

The first cases of HIV/AIDS recorded in Sydney, Australia, were in the late 1980s. Rates of infection increased into the early 1990s, but improvements in treatments in the mid 1990s coincided with stabilized rates of infection. At the end of 2001 there were an estimated 12 730 people living with HIV or AIDS in Australia and it is estimated that nationally 450 new HIV infections occur each year (National Centre in HIV Epidemiology and Clinical Research, 2002a). New South Wales accounts for around 60% of HIV and AIDS diagnoses in Australia (National Centre in HIV Epidemiology and Clinical Research, 2002b) and at the end of September 2002 there were 9277 HIV-positive people in the state (National Centre in HIV Epidemiology and Clinical Research, 2003). There is some indication of a rise in the number of new HIV infections in Australia in 2003, although firm epidemiological data are limited at this time (National Centre in HIV Epidemiology and Clinical Research, 2002b).

Prior to 1996, with limited treatment options, a diagnosis of HIV generally meant death, possibly within months, almost certainly within years. As the illness progressed and function decreased, people living with HIV or AIDS became more dependent on others and on the numerous statutory and voluntary HIV services available. These services operated from a palliative care perspective and were designed to provide short periods of intense assistance to people who were dying (Yallop, 2000).

In mid-1996, significant changes occurred in the treatment of HIV and AIDS. The advent of highly active anti-retroviral therapies, involving new combinations of three or four anti-HIV drugs, greatly reduced the levels of HIV detectable in the blood, and for many people this meant a dramatic improvement in health. For those newly diagnosed with HIV, these drugs brought a new sense of hope for the future. The introduction of these treatments has been a major milestone in the medical treatment of HIV and AIDS. As this change in treatments and therapies has developed, enhancing life expectancy, some have speculated that HIV has now become a long-term chronic condition rather than an acute life threatening illness (Lowth *et al.*, 1999).

The changes in medication regimens were initially hailed as a cure, but this is not the case. While many people continue to respond to these treatments and are enjoying better levels of health, the long-term benefits of these medications are not known. There is, nevertheless, a new sense of energy and hope that did not previously exist (Cohen, 1997; Hay, 1997; Odets, 1997). Interestingly, the changes are not always welcomed, as the future is an uncertain one. Tuller (1996, p. 7) describes this as 'uncertain life after certain death' and describes it as 'the struggle between the self who yearns for a return to life and the self who has accepted impending death'.

It is also clear now that there are many side efffects associated with the drugs, and that not all people living with HIV or AIDS are responding to the medications. The issue of compliance with medication regimens is also a complex one (Nelmes, 1997; Lowth *et al.*, 1999), with many people expected to take large numbers of pills each day for the rest of their life. So, although these recent changes in HIV care have brought optimism, they have also brought many complex issues and challenges for those with the virus and those involved in providing services for people living with HIV (Tuller, 1996; Nelmes, 1997; Odets, 1997).

There has been some research describing the resulting issues of this changing context for people living with HIV or AIDS (e.g. Ezzy *et al.*, 1998; Brashers *et al.*, 1999; Lowth *et al.*, 1999). This new context challenges many people living with HIV or AIDS to reconstruct a future which they never thought existed. This can mean attempting to establish new relationships, dealing with long-term financial debt, considering returning to employment and facing the idea of having to comply with medication regimens for the foreseeable future. These changes prompt an identity change from a person with an acute life-threatening illness to someone with a long-term chronic condition.

10.2.1   Impact on occupation

This changing context has also had a significant impact on the self-maintenance, productivity and leisure occupations of many people living with HIV and AIDS. In the late 1980s and early 1990s many people living with HIV and AIDS, expecting to die within years, restructured their lives. This often involved an occupational shift as emphasis was placed on occupations that were most important and meaningful as they faced imminent death. For example, in order to have some quality of life many people abandoned major work roles to travel or devote more time to family and friends. For some, being HIV-positive became the centre of their occupational performance and the majority of their occupations became centred around HIV. Time was spent attending medical appointments, seeing counsellors, dealing with government-funded social services, attending HIV peer support groups and social functions, being a volunteer for AIDS organizations and caring for friends who were at the end stages of AIDS. Being HIV-positive was the major productivity role (Yallop, 1999). Dessaix (1996, p. 195) describes his personal experience of this phenomenon:

> 'One or two of the men seem to live totally for being ill: Monday – gym, Tuesday – action committee, Wednesday – gym, Thursday – hydrotherapy, Friday – newsletter. Being ill gives meaning to everything, it's at the heart of every conversation, it's the reason for having breakfast and turning the key to start the car. It's as if life lived without this disease would lose all its gravity and significance.'

However, as function reduced as the illness progressed, these occupations were replaced by tasks associated with dying, such as creating a will, saying goodbye to family and contemplating spiritual issues. As with other conditions treated palliatively, the ability to engage in previously satisfying occupations was limited by declining physical function (van der Ploeg, 2001).

The current situation for many people living with HIV and AIDS is somewhat different and concerns about death and illness are no longer as central (Roy & Cain, 2001). The improved health that many people living with HIV gained due to the developments in treatments resulted in an occupational dilemma. Those who were forced to reduce their occupations due to increasing illness suddenly faced being physically well enough to engage in more occupations than in the past. The occupations associated with being ill were no longer relevant and left many people living with HIV and AIDS feeling bored, isolated and with a new sense of time and energy not previously experienced. While physical health had improved for many, this did not necessarily correspond with improvements in emotional, spiritual and psychological health. People living with HIV and AIDS still struggle with many other health issues including social isolation, poverty, grief, loss and ongoing uncertainty (Brashers *et al.*, 1999; Trainor & Ezer, 2000). The changing context of HIV left many people living with HIV and AIDS occupationally deprived, particularly in relation to productive occupations. This changing context also prompts a reconsideration of the future, and a shift from preparing for death to living with HIV. This can be a difficult and complex process, in a way more challenging than death, which seemed to be definite, certain and expected. These issues make the process of reconstructing and redeveloping new occupations all the more challenging (Brashers *et al.*, 1999; Trainor & Ezer, 2000).

Reconstructing productive occupations can also force people living with HIV and AIDS to confront breaking away from a welfare support model. The response to the emergence of HIV in Sydney was strong and swift, and many welfare, food, financial and housing services were established to maximize the quality of life of terminally ill people. The focus has now shifted and HIV services no longer have the funding necessary to continue this level of long-term support. There are still people living with HIV and AIDS who require crisis and welfare assistance but there are also many who have become dependent on these services, a situation which cannot be maintained in the long term. HIV service providers and the relevance of their services are also challenged (Lowth *et al.*, 1999; Yallop *et al.*, 2002).

Some people living with HIV and AIDS and service providers are reluctant to surrender this model of service provision, as it fulfils need on both parts. There are benefits for people living with HIV and AIDS remaining in a 'sick' role, such as support and attention. There are also difficulties, however, such as being labelled and marginalized and losing a sense of independence and self-responsibility. Embracing wellness means relinquishing some of the attention and importance associated with being sick or dying. This can be a very challenging process as many people living with HIV and AIDS, as described above, have been involved with services for so long that it has become a way of life.

For the purposes of this chapter the process described above, of redeveloping meaningful occupational roles prompted by increasing health, is termed 'occupational reconstruction'. As part of this occupational reconstruction process a number of people living with HIV and AIDS are contemplating the redevelopment of a productivity role, specifically returning to paid employment.

10.2.2   Employment issues for people living with HIV and AIDS

Returning to work has many benefits for people living with HIV and AIDS, including financial reward, increased social contact, structure and routine through occupation, involvement in meaningful activity, being able to contribute to society and help others, increased self-esteem and confidence, better use of time and a reason for getting up in the morning (Yallop, 2000; McReynolds, 2001). In short, becoming involved in productive occupation again gives a reason for living and it gives meaning and identity beyond that of being HIV-positive.

The benefits associated with returning to paid work are attractive, but the decision to return to paid work is complex and can be overwhelming. It is also only one of many aspects of reconstructing a future orientation. Returning to work raises issues such as adjusting to a focus on living rather than dying, financial issues including the loss of benefits, fluctuations in health, complex medication regimens to be taken during work time, disclosure and discrimination, explaining periods out of the workforce, lost confidence and self-esteem, uncertainty of the long-term benefits of HIV medications and care, and a common desire to change career paths, often, because values have changed through the process of living with HIV (Yallop, 2000; Salz, 2001). Many people living with HIV and AIDS describe feeling pressured by a society that strongly links identity and worth to being engaged in paid work. Some grapple with the genuine desire to work and reap the benefits and the fear that it may have a negative impact on their health (Crockett, 1997). This can be more complex in countries where health benefits are dependent on employment.

An added complexity is the changed life perspective that many people living with HIV and AIDS describe after having been so close to death and been given a chance at life again. For some, this experience has altered their sense of what is important to achieve in life, what activities are sources of meaningful engagement in the world and what are worthwhile ways in which to expend energy and time. A shifting focus from preparing for death to imagining new possibilities in life has a profound impact on some individuals (Brashers *et al.*, 1999).

10.2.3   Positive Employment Service

Positive Employment Service (PES) is an occupational therapy service developed in 1997 in direct response to the changed HIV context. Overall, PES aims to enhance quality of life, well-being and health for people living with HIV and AIDS by addressing issues related to productive occupations (see Table 10.1). The service supports people living with HIV and AIDS who are seeking a change in their work situation and assists them to explore future work options, make informed choices and decisions about those options and reconstruct productivity roles. The changes that clients might explore include returning to work, changing current work or becoming more productive without paid employment. The service has a focus on productive occupations but is not limited to paid

Table 10.1   Positive Employment Service aim and objectives.

Aim
- To enhance quality of life, well-being and health for people with HIV and AIDS by addressing issues of employment.

Objectives
- People living with HIV and AIDS will increase their awareness of information, options and resources related to work.
- People living with HIV and AIDS will identify their own needs and abilities and increase their self-awareness related to working.
- People living with HIV and AIDS will make their informed choices and create their own goals about employment and work.
- People living with HIV and AIDS will be linked to vocational and avocational services appropriate to their needs.

employment. PES recognizes that work takes different forms for different people (paid work, study, training, volunteer work, development of an interest) and the emphasis is on finding personally meaningful occupations.

PES also aims to impact indirectly on health by working in partnership with HIV, health and employment related organizations, to shape policy and create supportive environments for people living with HIV and AIDS to explore and engage in productive activity. Examples of this include involvement in developing work trial programmes within HIV organizations, assessing the impact of government welfare reforms on people living with HIV and AIDS and addressing workplace discrimination through employer education.

Because the aims of PES are related to the broader notion of productive occupation rather than just paid employment, outcomes for the service relate to participants' engagement in productive occupations and a process of self-development. These contrast many government-funded employment services that focus on the outcome of gaining training or paid employment. While this is appropriate for some people living with HIV and AIDS, and certainly some have benefited from involvement with these services, the focus on the outcome of paid work excludes, and is not relevant to, many people living with HIV and AIDS. To date PES clients have expressed a strong need for time to contemplate their situation, assess the realistic options and discuss strategies and goals for the future. This process needs to occur prior to even considering paid work and can take months. For some people living with HIV and AIDS the outcome of paid employment is also not realistic or desired, but there may still be a need for assistance to develop other kinds of occupational roles.

10.3   Establishing client need

A number of theoretical models were used in the development of PES and continue to guide assessment and intervention. These included occupational therapy models such as the Canadian Model of Occupational Performance (Canadian Association of Occupational Therapists, 1997) and Kielhofner's (1995) Model of Human Occupation. Vocational rehabilitation models such as Choose Get Keep (Anthony *et al.*, 1984) and Stevens' (1995) Model of Career Development are also drawn upon in providing the PES service. Due to the unique nature of the service no one model is appropriate and a blend of approaches is used during interactions with clients.

The PES assessment process occurs through the use of informal interviews. The initial session starts with an introduction to occupational therapy and the PES service, including an explanation of the aims and objectives of the service. The therapist also provides a description of the usual PES client process and possible outcomes of the client-therapist relationship. It is important that at this time the therapist emphasizes the client centred nature of PES. PES is based on a belief that the client is the expert about their issues and experiences, while the therapist acts as a guide and coach.

The first step in establishing client need is to identify the client's motivation for approaching the service. This can be partly uncovered by discussing the method of referral to the service. The majority of clients become aware of PES through word of mouth and regular publicity and are self-referred. Clients are also referred by other health and HIV community workers and a small number are referred by other government employment agencies. An important exercise completed with PES clients in the initial interview assists to identify intrinsic and extrinsic factors affecting their desire for occupational change. These factors are categorized into factors that motivate change and factors that create barriers to change. Table 10.2 lists some examples of factors identified by PES clients. The identification of these factors influences how the therapist approaches the client interaction. It is important within the therapy process to utilize the motivating factors to encourage clients along the change process and work with clients to develop strategies of dealing with the perceived barriers.

Table 10.2 Motivators of and barriers to change.

	Intrinsic factors	Extrinsic factors
Motivators	• Desire to earn money • Desire to develop new social networks • Desire to develop new skills • Desire to contribute to society	• Lack of social status of unemployment • Lack of activity leading to boredom
Barriers	• Low self-esteem and confidence • Uncertainty about ability to return to work	• Fluctuating health • Side effects of medications • Lack of support • Lack of skills and training • Age

The next important issue to explore in the assessment process is the occupational change sought by the client. At this point it may be helpful for the therapist to elaborate further on the broader meaning of the term occupation, in relation to all purposeful activity. It is also important to explain that the focus of PES is on productive occupation and not only paid employment. Information about the occupational change the client is seeking can be uncovered by discussing what prompted the client to approach the service. Further exploration occurs through assessment of current occupations. Most importantly, it is essential to explore how the client would like their occupations to be different. The following questions can be used to assist the unfolding of this process:

• Describe a typical day (may be appropriate to give the client a weekly timetable to fill in and bring to the next session).
• What routines are important to you?

- What activities do you need, want and choose to do?
- How has this occupational performance changed over time and what has been the impact of living with HIV on your occupations?
- How would you like your occupational performance to be different in the future?
- Why are you looking for this change at this time in your life? Why now and not earlier?

The third step in the PES assessment process refines the discussion to the specific area of productivity. At this stage it is appropriate to discuss past, present and future productivity roles, including, if appropriate, an employment history. It is essential that the client has a clear understanding of the notion of occupation and the PES definition of work encompassing more than paid employment. At times clients raise occupational issues related to self-care or leisure. If it becomes clear at this point that a client wants to work on occupational goals not related to productive activity, referrals can be made to other community based health professionals, including occupational therapists, and relevant services. At times it is difficult to classify productive in contrast to non-productive occupational goals and this needs to be assessed on an individual basis. This stage of the assessment is an opportunity to provide clients with education related to the theories of occupational therapy and occupational science in language that is appropriate and meaningful to the client.

Environmental considerations are also essential to explore within the assessment process. The physical environment, in particular having stable accommodation, is a priority before initiating occupational change. Assessment of the cultural environment provides important insights into work values and role expectations. The social environment is also a key factor; for example, whether the client has supportive family or friends who will be able to provide assistance during the process of occupational change. It is also important to explore strengths and resources, initially from the client's perspective, but this is also an opportunity for the therapist to provide feedback to the client on what they perceive to be the client's strengths and resources. These factors will assist the client most when the PES process of occupational change becomes challenging. Examples of strengths may include an optimistic outlook, an ability to communicate well or a very supportive friend.

10.3.1   A case study: Frank's assessment

To illustrate the assessment process, a summary of a PES assessment will be presented, using the areas outlined in the previous section.

Frank is a 42 year-old man living in inner Sydney in government-subsidized housing. Frank has been HIV-positive for 12 years and has been receiving a disability support pension for the past ten years. Two years after his diagnosis Frank became very unwell and so retired from work. He describes a number of HIV-related illnesses and hospitalizations, including one episode where he was given three months to live. Frank commenced HIV combination drug therapy two years prior to his initial contact with PES and his health improved as a result. Frank had a long history of alcohol and heroin use but he has been clean for six months. He attends weekly sessions with a counsellor which he finds very supportive. Frank had been in contact with PES previously but he ceased involvement as he was still struggling with drug and alcohol issues. Prior to being on a disability pension, Frank describes working in a variety of retail and sales positions, including work in a large department store.

Motivation

During the initial assessment process Frank identified several intrinsic and extrinsic motivators and barriers. The motivating factors included: desire to earn money and contribute to society (intrinsic); status of worker within his social network and boredom due to lack of occupation (extrinsic). The barriers he perceived included: decreased confidence about his appearance, due to HIV-related weight loss (intrinsic); fluctuating health, lack of skills and training, age, inconsistent work history (extrinsic).

Occupational change

When asked to describe a typical day, Frank responded:

'Get up at 10.00 am and have a light breakfast, meet friends for a coffee, attend lunch at the HIV support centre, have an afternoon sleep, meet with my counsellor, cook dinner, spend time on the Internet at night and go to bed at midnight.'

Frank was also asked about routines and occupations that were important to him:

'Meeting with my counsellor has been a very important and supportive aspect of my life over the past year. I still feel very dependent on this. I also really like the support I receive from the guys at the HIV centre as I don't have many other friends. Apart from that, I feel quite bored with my life at the moment and feel like I am just filling in spare time during the other parts of my day. I feel like I sleep too much ... and I feel like I have very little energy in the morning.'

Frank also reflected on how his occupational performance had changed over time and how HIV had impacted on his occupations:

'Before having HIV I used to be someone who was full of energy and always on the go. I loved my work in sales and was very successful. When I was first diagnosed I went into denial and continued with the same high energy lifestyle, but things caught up with me and I became very unwell. For ten years I feel like I have been on a roller coaster ride, not knowing how long I have left to live. My life was out of control when I was addicted to heroin and drinking all the time. I have had a little more hope over the last two years with my improved health due to HIV treatments. And even more hope now that I am off the drugs for good. The pneumonia has thrown me a little bit and I don't have much confidence but I want to make a new start with my life and do the things I have always dreamed about.'

When asked how he wanted his occupational performance to be different, Frank stated that he felt bored and felt that he did not contribute to wider society. He had a strong desire to find a job that he enjoyed and allowed him to earn enough money to support an enjoyable lifestyle. When asked why he felt the time was right to make these changes, Frank reflected:

'I tried to make a change through PES last year and feel embarrassed that it failed, it just wasn't the right time for me. I couldn't get myself together enough to get to appointments on time and I was still using drugs which made me feel awful physically and emotionally. I feel like I have really made some ground in the counselling sessions and I feel like I am really ready for a change now.'

Productive occupations

In the past, Frank's work history involved some sporadic work in retail and sales. He was dismissed from two positions for stealing to support his heroin addiction. He has a ten-year gap in his paid employment, due to HIV-related illnesses. At present Frank is enrolled on a computer course at the local HIV support centre and is finding this challenging as he has not used a computer for a number of years. He has also been studying for his driver's licence which lapsed a number of years ago, as he feels this will assist him in gaining work. Frank identified that he would like to become a real estate agent in the eastern suburbs of Sydney.

Environment

Frank lives in government-subsidized housing. He dislikes living there due to the chaotic lifestyle of many of his neighbours. A major motivator for returning to paid work is that it will enable him to move out of his current accommodation. Frank's parents are German and he speaks fluent German. Although his family moved here when he was very young he still feels a connection to Germany and has travelled there a number of times. Frank has very little contact with his family and has had numerous arguments with them about drug taking in the past, that have damaged relationships. Frank has a few good friends but lost many when he was using drugs. He feels very supported by the local HIV support centre and his counsellor.

Strengths and resources

Frank and the therapist identified the following strengths and resources:

- Frank looks younger than his age, which he thought might be useful when applying for jobs.

- Frank felt very supported by his counsellor.
- Frank felt he had a positive attitude towards making changes in his life.

10.4 Planning the occupational therapy intervention

The assessment process usually spans a number of sessions and at times is interspersed with actual interventions. The main assessment period is usually conducted in three one-hour sessions over a three-week period. Once the therapist has gained an understanding of attitude to change, occupational performance and specific productivity role performance, the occupational intervention can be planned.

PES clients use a goal planner to identify long-, medium- and short-term goals. It is important to note that people living with HIV and AIDS may define long term differently to other clients as they have faced a diagnosis of a terminal illness and will probably have an altered perspective of the future. It is essential to be aware of how far into the future a client is comfortable with planning, as many clients still have a sense of a limited lifespan. Long-term goal development is usually one, possibly two, years ahead. It is essential to be sensitive to this process of reconstructing a sense of future, given that it can be difficult. Medium-term goals may reach six months to one year into the future, while short-term goals will be achievable within a number of weeks or months, depending on the client.

This process can be challenging for the therapist at times, especially if there is a difference between what the client and therapist assess as a realistic and achievable goal. It is important to be reflective as a therapist and not impose rigid judgements about a client's capabilities. Years of professional experience may give insight into whether goals are realistic for clients but it is important to balance this with allowing a client to dream about what is possible for their future. Often, through the process of short-term goal attainment, clients adjust their sense of what is realistic in the longer term. Challenging the realism of long-term goals is probably not appropriate early in the therapeutic relationship, as rapport needs to be developed in order to challenge the client in this way. Regular goal review is essential throughout the PES interventions.

10.4.1 Frank's goals

During his initial interview, Frank stated that his long-term goal was to be the top real estate consultant in one of the wealthiest areas of Sydney, within one year. From my past five years experience developing and providing PES I doubted whether this was realistic due to a number of factors, including Frank's erratic work history, ten-year gap since paid employment, his prior struggles with drug addiction and currently fluctuating health. It was not appropriate to express these concerns to Frank as we had only started to develop rapport, so instead we discussed why the goal was so important and why he wanted to achieve it. Together Frank and I broke the long-term goal into achievable medium-term and short-term goals. Over the following weeks, through the process of achieving short-term goals and dealing with the associated challenges, Frank came to the realization that his long-term goal was unrealistic and not something he could achieve within the one- to two-year time frame. We used this insight to revisit and rewrite the long-term goal. Table 10.3 outlines some of the goals developed with Frank.

Table 10.3 Frank's goals

Short term
- I will update my curriculum vitae to be appropriate for applying for part-time sales positions by the next PES appointment.
- Over the next three PES appointments I will complete three vocational assessments and discuss the results with my therapist.
- I will investigate enrolling in a community college computer skills course and bring the information along to my next PES session to discuss.

Medium term
- In three months time I will be employed in a volunteer position within an HIV community organization to assist in developing my administration skills.
- In six months time I will be employed in a part-time administration position.

Long term
- In two years time I will be employed as a real estate agent.

10.5   Implementing the occupational therapy intervention

There are a number of ways of implementing the PES intervention depending on the goals set. Overall, PES intervention is aimed at assisting clients to make informed decisions about occupational change and assist them to enact that change. Some of the key PES interventions are briefly outlined below.

Occupational values/skills exploration

- Commonly used with clients who have spent some time out of the workforce and are looking to return to paid work.
- Clarifies what is valued in a work role, what skills the client has and needs, and identifies relevant fields of work.

Positive decisions programme

- Three-month work experience and training programme (including administration and marketing) for people living with HIV and AIDS developed by a community HIV organization and PES.

- Enables clients to engage in new occupational roles within a safe and supported environment with no concerns about disclosure of HIV status.
- PES provides ongoing support throughout the programme.

Volunteer work

- Often used as a training and transition time for clients who are not yet ready for paid work, but may also be an outcome for clients not wanting paid work.
- Volunteer work must be meaningful, supportive and enable the client to develop skills and confidence.
- Can be a good way of gaining references and developing networks within a certain industry.
- Non-threatening way for clients to self-assess their ability to cope in a work environment.

Skills development

- Appropriate for clients who do not have the skills necessary to enter their desired field of work. It is often required for those moving into a new work area.
- The study environment is often less pressured and formal than a work environment and therefore acts as a transition environment.
- PES intervention involves discussion of reasons for study, investigation of usefulness of study, discussing what the study will lead to, developing skills around the application process and ongoing support while in study.

Interest development

- Appropriate for clients who decide they do not want to aim for paid work and is common with clients who are unwell or approaching retirement age.
- PES intervention assists clients to assess their current occupational roles, explore interest areas and develop strategies to enhance their participation in new non-paid productive roles.

Job search support

- Provision of practical support and skills development related to the search for paid work. This may include developing a curriculum vitae, interview skills and negotiating government-funded social security and employment services.
- PES draws on career counselling and vocational rehabilitation models in the provision of these services.

Group programmes

- Peer support is an important aspect of the PES process.
- There are a number of support groups for people living with HIV and AIDS

which address issues of life reconstruction, including the development of productive activity.
- PES facilitates sessions related to work issues in a number of these group programmes.

Self employment

- Appropriate for clients wanting to develop opportunities for self employment.
- PES interventions include identifying interest areas for self employment, information gathering and referral to specialist self employment services.

Life coaching

- PES has connections with a recently developed HIV coaching service which can assist clients to develop and achieve broader life goals.

10.5.1   Occupational therapy interventions for Frank

Occupational values/skills exploration

This intervention was selected as Frank had spent ten years out of paid employment and expressed some uncertainty about his skills and interests. Frank's long-term goal was related to returning to paid work and developing a career path and so these vocational assessments were highly appropriate. Three PES sessions were spent exploring work skills and values using standard career assessments, such as the Career Values Card Sort (Knowdell, 1989) and the Motivated Skills Card Sort (Knowdell, 1990). The results from these assessments prompted discussion and reflection about appropriate future work choices and enabled Frank to confirm that he was suited to administration and sales work.

Volunteer work

This intervention was also selected due to Frank's ten-year gap in employment and desire to return to paid work. Frank saw this as an appropriate first step to redevelop his administration skills and work stamina. PES has developed a network with a range of HIV community organizations providing volunteer programmes. Using the results of the work values and skills assessments, Frank and the therapist selected an appropriate volunteer position as an administration assistant at an HIV community centre. PES assisted in liaising with the manager of the centre and provided ongoing support to Frank while he was volunteering. Due to his decreased work stamina, Frank started his position one day a week and increased this to two days a week one month later.

Job search support

One month after Frank had commenced volunteer work, with the assistance of PES, he started to explore the idea of returning to paid employment. He developed a curriculum vitae appropriate for administration positions and was able to include his volunteer position as recent experience. Time was spent exploring how to explain the ten-year gap in his employment history and Frank decided to include a number of unpaid and cash-in-hand positions to cover this period. Time was also spent discussing the issue of disclosing his HIV status in his curriculum vitae, in an interview, and once in employment. Frank was provided with PES fact sheets and information from the Anti-Discrimination Board to supplement these discussions and assist him with making informed choices about disclosure. PES also provided Frank with a practice interview to assist in preparation for job searching.

10.6 Evaluation and discharge

The PES process involves continual evaluation as it is essential to re-evaluate goals set to ensure the ongoing relevance and value of the service. The length of time involved with the service varies with individual clients and there is no imposed timeframe for discharge. Some clients only require a few sessions, while others are involved with the service over a number of years. The therapist needs to use professional and clinical judgement to negotiate appropriate cessation of services with the client. Goal attainment is obviously one indicator that can be used to help make decisions about discharge. The final session is used as a review of the occupational change that has occurred through PES. Goals are reviewed and, if relevant, a plan of follow-up support is determined. This may include a follow-up telephone call, email or just an agreement that the client will contact PES if further support is required. This session is important in providing closure for both therapist and client.

The use of formal outcome tools has been an ongoing challenge as it has been difficult to find a tool that measures relevant and appropriate indicators. Many employment related services monitor client outcomes using indicators such as numbers entering formal training or paid employment. These indicators do not recognize less concrete outcomes that measure the distance travelled towards occupational change and are therefore not appropriate or relevant to PES clients. PES has had some success using the Rickter Scale (Hutchinson & Stead, 1994), an assessment tool developed in the UK which measures the distance travelled towards employability. It is a self-report tool which measures changes in items such as confidence with decision making about work, self-esteem, readiness for work and practical work skills.

10.6.1   Evaluation and discharge of Frank

Frank remained in contact with PES for one year. During this time he gained an understanding of his work values and skills, developed his curriculum vitae, practised his interview skills, completed a basic course in information technology and the Internet, held a volunteer administration position for six months and obtained a part-time administration position in a homewares store. During the initial assessment phase Frank attended weekly PES sessions, but as time progressed the PES sessions became fortnightly and then monthly. Support was provided during the first two months of his paid position and at this point both Frank and the therapist felt regular PES sessions were no longer required. Frank still has a long-term goal of studying for and being employed as a real estate agent. Frank knows that he can always access phone or face-to-face support from PES in the future, as required.

10.7   Conclusion

Health care for people living with HIV and AIDS has changed dramatically since 1996. The introduction of HIV combination treatments and resulting improvements in health has created an occupational dilemma for many. With a renewed sense of energy and time, but limited occupational roles, many people living with HIV and AIDS feel bored, isolated and occupationally deprived. Occupational therapists have an important and unique role to play in assisting people living with HIV and AIDS to dream, explore, choose and organize occupations as part of the complex process of occupational reconstruction. Positive Employment Service has been specifically developed to assist with reconstructing productive occupation. PES has assisted over 600 people living with HIV and AIDS over the past seven years. The uniqueness of the service lies in its emphasis on occupational reconstruction, which enables people living with HIV and AIDS to develop a renewed sense of self, life meaning and potential. Frank's summary:

> 'PES has helped restore the sense of myself and I have started to go out and engage in other activities in a range of ways, instead of sitting in front of the TV. Through PES I feel like I have come back to life again.'

References

Anthony, W.A., Howell, J. & Danley, K. (1984). Vocational rehabilitation of the psychiatrically disabled. In: M. Mirabi (Ed.), *The Chronically Mentally Ill: Research and Services* (pp. 215–237). New York: Spectrum Publications.

Brashers, D., Neidig, J., Cardillo, L., Dobbs, L., Russell, J. & Haas, S. (1999). In an important way I did die: uncertainty and revival in persons living with HIV or AIDS. *AIDS Care, 11* (2), 201–219.

Canadian Association of Occupational Therapists (1997). *Enabling Occupation: an Occupational Therapy Perspective.* Ottawa: CAOT Publications.

Cohen, J. (1997). The media's love affair with AIDS research: Hope vs hype. *Science, 275,* 298–299.

Crockett, P. (1997). So you're thinking about going back to work. Retrieved 15 May, 2003 from http://www.thebody.com/crockett/bk2work.html

Dessaix, R. (1996). *Night Letters.* Sydney: Pan Macmillan

Ezzy, D., de Visser, R., Bartos, M., McDonald, K., O'Donnell, D. & Rosenthal, D. (1998). *HIV Futures Community Report: Health, Relationships, Community and Employment.* Melbourne: National Centre in HIV Social Research, La Trobe University.

Hay, D. (1997). Hope in the time of AIDS. *Sydney Morning Herald Good Weekend Magazine,* 22 March, 42–46.

Hutchinson, R. & Stead, K. (1994). *The Rickter Scale.* Inverness: The Rickter Company Ltd.

Kielhofner, G. (1995). *A Model of Human Occupation: Theory and Application.* Baltimore: Williams & Wilkins.

Knowdell, R. (1989). *Career Values Card Sort.* California: Career Research and Testing Inc.

Knowdell, R. (1990). *Motivated Skills Card Sort.* California: Career Research and Testing Inc.

Lowth, A.,Yallop, S., Reid, J. & Fitzgerald, M.H. (1999). Looking beyond the optimism surrounding new treatments: issues for HIV service providers and people living with HIV. *Australian Social Work, 52* (3), 28–33.

McReynolds, C. (2001). The meaning of work in the lives of people living with HIV disease and AIDS. *Rehabilitation Counselling Bulletin, 44* (2), 104–115.

National Centre in HIV Epidemiology and Clinical Research (2002a). *HIV/AIDS, Viral Hepatitis and Sexually Transmissible Infections in Australia Annual Surveillance Report 2002.* Sydney: National Centre in HIV Epidemiology and Clinical Research.

National Centre in HIV Epidemiology and Clinical Research (2002b). *Australian HIV Surveillance Report, 18* (4). Sydney: National Centre in HIV Epidemiology and Clinical Research.

National Centre in HIV Epidemiology and Clinical Research. (2003). *Australian HIV Surveillance Report, 19* (1). Sydney: National Centre in HIV Epidemiology and Clinical Research.

Nelmes, P. (1997). Elation and devastation. *Talkabout,* 11 August, 10–11.

Odets, W. (1997). Hope against hope. *POZ Magazine, 47,* 71–72.

van der Ploeg, W. (2001). Health promotion in palliative care: an occupational perspective. *Australian Occupational Therapy Journal, 48* (1), 45–48.

Roy, C. & Cain, R. (2001). The involvement of people living with HIV/AIDS in community-based organizations: contributions and constraints. *AIDS Care, 13* (4), 421–432.

Salz, F. (2001). HIV/AIDS and work: the implications for occupational therapy. *Work, 16* (3), 269–272.

Stevens, P. (1995). *Model of Career Development.* Sydney: Worklife Pty Ltd.

Trainor, A. & Ezer, H. (2000). Rebuilding life: the experience of living with AIDS after facing imminent death. *Qualitative Health Research, 10* (5), 646–660.

Tuller, D. (1996). Uncertain life after certain death. *San Francisco Chronicle,* 24 November, 1.

Yallop, S. (1999). Positive employment service – facilitating employment for people living with HIV. *Work, 13,* 211–215.

Yallop, S. (2000). Identity issues for people living with HIV/AIDS: humans with potential or sexual victims? *British Journal of Occupational Therapy*, *63* (9), 419–424.

Yallop, S., Lowth, A., Fitzgerald, M.H., Reid, J. & Morelli, A. (2002). The changing world of HIV care: the impact on health professionals. *Culture, Health and Sexuality*, *4* (4), 431–441.

Chapter 11
Therapeutic Occupation Following Stroke: A Case Study

Janet Golledge

11.1   Introduction

At the end of this chapter the reader will appreciate that the therapeutic application of occupation is essential for enabling functional recovery following a stroke. The importance of an understanding of neuroplasticity, motor learning and promoting generalization of learning will be highlighted. These concepts are fundamental to effective therapy and for facilitating engagement in occupation. A case study of Harry (a pseudonym), will be used to illustrate intervention. Although the initial hospital based phase will be explained to set the scene, the majority of Harry's contact with occupational therapy occurred when he was discharged home. These community based therapy sessions will reflect my input as a member of the team and my use of occupations with Harry. The importance of working holistically will be stressed. Superficially, Harry had a physical disability following a stroke but the emotional consequences were equally significant. It is essential that occupational therapists deal with the sadness and pain of individuals' experiences as well as the more readily observed aspects. It is not the aim of this chapter to explain the neuroanatomy and neurophysiology of stroke or intervention from other health professionals. The reader should identify additional texts for this information.

11.2   Overview: stroke and occupational therapy

A stroke is usually defined as 'a clinical syndrome typified by rapidly developing signs of focal or global disturbance of cerebral functions, lasting more than 24 hours or leading to death, with no apparent causes other than of vascular origin' (World Health Organization, 1980, cited in Rudd *et al.*, 1999, p. 5). Strokes are most commonly associated with older individuals but younger adults can also experience a stroke. It involves the interruption of the blood supply to part of the brain, usually a cerebral hemisphere of the brain or in the brain stem. They are the third most common cause of death in the UK and other developed countries, with approximately 30% of people dying in the month after a stroke (Stephen & Rafferty, 1994; Department of Health, 2001). A stroke is also the greatest cause of severe disability, as although 65% of survivors live independently, 35% of all survivors are significantly disabled and are likely to require considerable help with daily occupations (Stephen & Rafferty, 1994; Department of Health, 2001). As a result, a substantial proportion of health and social care resources are devoted to the immediate and continuing care of people following a stroke (Wolf *et al.*, 1996).

The consequences of a stroke are extremely varied and may include difficulties in motor ability, perceptual-cognitive skills, emotional reactions and social functioning. Although viewing the impact of a stroke in this way helps to clarify the impairments for each individual and provide a consistent terminology for different health team members, they reflect a biomedical focus. A stroke is a revolutionary event that interrupts the continuity of the individual's journey through life. Focusing on impairments does not sufficiently reflect the enormity of the consequences for individuals. Occupational therapists look beyond these impairments and analyse the impact of an individual's specific pattern of component problems on occupational performance. For example, hypertonia in flexor muscles of the upper limb might impact on occupations such as putting on shoes. Visual processing deficits might cause problems finding items in the fridge, putting the lid on a jar or correctly orienting clothes to the body. Dysphasia can significantly limit participation in conversation with others, listening to the radio, watching television, answering the telephone or accessing the Internet. These examples represent a fraction of the potential occupations influenced by just a few selected impairments.

Individuals who have had a stroke are referred to occupational therapists because they have some level of difficulty performing occupations. They are not referred because they cannot complete remedial games, stack cones, roll therapeutic putty or any other non-familiar activity (Golledge, 1998). During intervention occupational therapists should aim to find client centred, satisfying solutions to occupational difficulties so that individuals can begin to resume meaningful roles and provide purpose to engage in a lifestyle. Therapeutic use of occupation is vital for assisting individuals to begin and continue their process of adaptation, in helping them to make meaning of their lives (Forsberg-Warleby & Moller, 1996; Yerxa, 1998). Occupational therapists must ensure that an occupational focus guides their interventions with clients. This occupational perspective is the profession's unique contribution to supporting and enhancing the health of our clients (Johnson, 1996; Fisher, 1998; Wilcock, 1998; Yerxa, 1998). As this chapter progresses, the reader will appreciate that this occupational focus reflects research which highlights that recovery is best facilitated by helping individuals to engage in occupations that are meaningful and purposeful.

11.3   Harry: occupational deprivation after stroke

Harry was 58 years old when he had a stroke in his right cerebral hemisphere in September 2000. He was at home preparing to play golf the next day when, without warning, he fell onto the floor next to his golf bag. Golf balls rolled across the floor and Harry was not able to pick them up. He soon realized that he could not move his left arm or leg. Harry then felt an overwhelming urge to climb the stairs that were just in front of him so he dragged himself up the stairs, pushing with his right foot and pulling with his right hand. His wife found him struggling up the stairs and, concerned that he might have had a stroke, called for an ambulance.

Harry was admitted to the local hospital where he received medical care to stabilize his condition and identify the cause of his stroke: a cerebral infarction in the right internal capsule. Two days after admission to hospital Harry met the occupational therapist, Rose (a pseudonym). The initial interview involved Rose providing an explanation of occupational therapy and Harry sharing the story of his stroke and life before it.

Harry had been employed as a civil engineer, a job that involved travelling to various locations around the country. The job was physically and psychologically demanding and included monitoring a workforce and being responsible for time management and quality issues. Harry enjoyed his job but found the travelling tiring. His main leisure pursuit was playing golf and he also enjoyed gardening, DIY and socializing with his wife and friends. His wife, who had multiple sclerosis, completed all household domestic tasks. The couple had two adult daughters who they saw regularly.

11.3.1   Assessment

Rose completed a range of assessments to confirm the problems that Harry had as a result of his stroke and to establish a baseline against which future progress and final outcomes could be measured (see Table 11.1 for the assessments completed). Occupation based assessments were used as much as possible to help Harry understand the nature of occupational therapy and how Rose would engage him in the process of achieving valued occupational outcomes (Hocking, 2001). Self-care and productivity occupations were used for functional assessments. In this top-down approach, underlying components contributing to his functional difficulties were analysed subsequently.

Harry was anxious but cooperative with all assessments. He explained that he was left handed and wanted to regain as much function as possible, so that he could return to work and play golf. At the time of the assessment Harry was unable to complete any occupations independently and he needed assistance to stand and complete all transfers. While sitting in a wheelchair, he was able to retrieve items from the fridge, select cutlery and crockery. He could pour juice from a carton into a glass and pour cereal and milk into a bowl. Harry used only

Table 11.1   Assessments completed

- Behavioural Inattention Test (Wilson *et al.*, 1987)
- Rivermead Perceptual Assessment Battery (Whiting *et al.*, 1985)
- Barthel Index (Mahoney & Barthel, 1965)
- Non-standardized structured observations of Harry completing simple kitchen based occupations
- Non-standardized sensory assessment
- Non-standardized motor (specifically muscle tone) assessment
- Non-standardized assessment of emotional state

---

his right hand for all cutlery, which made cutting food difficult and necessitated swapping cutlery to eat. Harry was unable to write with his non-dominant right hand but could read books and the newspaper. The underlying component deficits which contributed to these occupational difficulties included hypotonia in muscles on the left side of his body, impaired balance and coordination, impaired sensory feedback in his left arm and leg, reduced motor control, and visual motor processing difficulties.

Emotionally, Harry was angry as he felt he had drawn the 'short straw'. His wife was becoming increasingly disabled and one of his daughters had some learning difficulties. It was clear that Harry needed opportunities within occupational therapy to explore his anger and feelings of emotional pain. His anger at the unfairness of life and the upset due to the loss of his most cherished occupations (work and golf) continued to be issues for Harry, and affected his relationship with his wife.

11.3.2   Planning intervention

Effective planning involves selection of relevant therapy approaches. Reflecting occupational therapy philosophy, these should be client centred, rather than profession centred. Rather than adapt to his difficulties, Harry wanted to regain as much of his prior function as possible. This suggested that remedial, rather than compensatory, therapy approaches would be most beneficial. To facilitate more effective movement in occupations, the Bobath concept was employed. The Bobath concept is a problem-solving approach to the assessment and treatment of individuals with disturbances of tone, movement and function due to a lesion of the central nervous system (CNS) (Lennon *et al.*, 2001; Panturin, 2001). Principles of motor learning were employed alongside this concept to facilitate engagement in occupations. The multicontext therapy approach, with its attention to promoting transfer of learning and generalization (Toglia, 1991; Toglia, 1998; Lee *et al.*, 2001), was also utilized to address his visual motor processing difficulties and ensure Harry did not merely rote learn specific occupations.

Neuroplasticity, motor learning and generalization: theory underpinning practice

A full consideration of the complex and fascinating topic of neuroplasticity is beyond the scope of this chapter, but a brief overview of salient aspects is presented.

Neuroplasticity is a term usually used to explain the capacity for structural reorganization and repair that can occur following injury to the CNS (Goldman & Plum, 1997; Ances & D'Esposito, 2000; Levin & Grafman, 2000; Selzer, 2000; Bach-y-Rita, 2001). The CNS is not a static structure but is constantly being reshaped according to environmental demands and needs. This reshaping occurs throughout life and includes the many mechanisms associated with learning, development and recovery from damage (Leonard, 1998). Since the demands made on the CNS will influence its structure, assisting clients to perform occupations will influence neuroplastic changes and so support future function (Johannsson, 2000; Liepert *et al.*, 2000; Bach-y-Rita, 2001; Cramer *et al.*, 2001). The therapeutic value of assisting clients to complete meaningful occupations as opposed to non-meaningful activities is supported by much research (Chollet *et al.*, 1991; Van Vliet *et al.*, 1995; Nelson *et al.*, 1996; Dean & Shepherd, 1997; Goldman & Plum, 1997; Wu *et al.*, 1998; Dolecheck & Schkade, 1999; Hochstenbach & Mulder, 1999; Rice *et al.*, 1999; Heddings *et al.*, 2000; Bach-y-Rita, 2001; Cramer *et al.*, 2001; Fisher & Sullivan, 2001; Unsworth & Cunningham, 2002).

Motor learning encompasses a range of different theories used to explain the acquisition and modification of motor behaviour (Shumway-Cook & Woollacott, 2001). For individuals following a stroke, motor learning is the process of re-acquiring the capability for skilled action, producing permanent changes in behaviour. The aim is to help individuals generalize or at least transfer their learning by attending to learning variables and feedback (Mathiowetz & Bass Haugen, 1994; Giuffrida, 1998; Sabari, 1998; Toglia, 1998).

Learning is a process mediated by the brain, in which the brain interprets and relates external sensory impressions with internally stored concepts. This system works most effectively when information or occupations to be learned are meaningful to the individual (Neistadt, 1998; Lee *et al.*, 2001). Following a stroke, errors in the information processing system can lead to difficulties performing occupations. Transfer of learning allows individuals to appreciate similarities between closely related tasks completed in familiar environments, using familiar equipment. Generalization is the ability to apply skills and problem-solving strategies learned in one situation to new situations, that is, transferring learning between different environments and occupations. This enables humans to effectively utilize learning gained from life experience.

11.3.3 Implementing intervention

Hospital facilities offer limited opportunities to complete occupations and are quite impoverished environments for individuals following a stroke. Occupations are decontextualized and environmental aspects are known to be a particularly crucial aspect for effective therapy (Head & Patterson, 1997; Brockman-Rubio, 1998; Ma *et al.*, 1999). Despite this, after six weeks in hospital Harry regained the ability to shower, groom, and dress himself independently. He was also able to transfer from chairs, the car and toilet, and walk with the aid of a stick. In the kitchen, he was able to make an instant drink and wash dishes. In contrast to hospital, an individual's home, work, leisure and social environments provide many rich and diverse opportunities for therapy. The remainder of this section will focus on occupational therapy Harry received after he had been discharged home. I visited Harry most weeks for nine months for treatment sessions. In addition, Harry had weekly sessions with an occupational therapy assistant and a physiotherapist for the six months following discharge from hospital.

Prior to my involvement another occupational therapist on the community team had used the Nottingham Extended Activities of Daily Living (NEADL) assessment (Nouri & Lincoln, 1987) and goal identification, in order to help identify Harry's priorities for occupational therapy. Harry's five goals were:

- To feed himself without help.
- To make a hot snack.
- To bend down and pick items off the floor with his right hand, e.g. golf balls, clothing, the post.
- To reach out and grip an object with his left hand, e.g. food from the fridge, door handles, his coat from a peg.
- To hold a golf club with his left and right hand whilst playing golf.

During my first session with Harry we talked about his life before the stroke, including his job and family. I wanted to ensure that I had a clear understanding of his current roles and those he wished to regain. It became clear that Harry had relinquished his employment role with great sadness, after acknowledging that he would not be able to cope with the physical demands of the job. We discussed his desire to contribute to general household chores, particularly as his wife was finding these increasingly fatiguing due to her multiple sclerosis. We explored what this might involve, what he felt able to do and how he wanted to achieve them.

It was clear that Harry was keen to use both upper limbs in the completion of occupations. Harry explained that his arm felt weak and that it required a lot of effort to move. He was aware that he was increasingly only using his right arm to complete occupations because it was easier, less time consuming and not as tiring. He confirmed that he wanted to use his left arm and not be so reliant on the right arm. I suggested that we continue using the Bobath concept to facilitate movement in his trunk and left upper and lower limbs. Prior to his stroke, Harry regularly mowed the front lawn and kept the back patio tidy and he wanted to continue with these occupations. Harry was very keen to return to his local golf course to play golf, but also, importantly, to socialize with friends. In addition to golf, prior to his stroke Harry had used a range of home exercise equipment to help maintain his physical fitness. Since returning home he had continued using some of this to increase strength in his lower limbs. He was keen to purchase other equipment to enable him to pursue this leisure interest. Harry also enjoyed reading books about history, but felt as though he spent 'too much time watching the television'. He wanted to relinquish this new habit but admitted he was avoiding productive occupations because he was dissatisfied with his efforts.

Based on the previous occupational therapy assessment and my own contact with Harry I saw the factors impacting on his ability to complete occupations to be:

- Moderate hypertonia had developed in prime mover muscles for shoulder girdle retraction, shoulder joint adduction and internal rotation, forearm pronation, wrist flexion and flexion for all digit joints.
- Subluxed left shoulder joint, with weak abduction and flexion, but no pain.
- Weak shoulder joint and elbow flexion and extension.
- Impaired dexterity in his left hand, weak power grip, and limited active digit extension.
- Difficulties with the spatio-temporal aspects of movement.

After discussion with Harry, we agreed to use a wide range of occupations in therapy sessions in order to achieve his goals and these are presented in Table 11.2. Harry also used therapy to understand his stroke, to talk about his feelings of anger and frustration and discuss his relationship with his wife.

Table 11.2 Occupations agreed upon for therapy.

- Washing dishes, putting shopping away, cleaning work surfaces, making drinks and snacks, tidy sitting and dining rooms, vacuum carpets, folding laundry
- Garden: mowing the lawn, moving the wheely bin each week for refuse collection, sweeping the path
- DIY projects: relocating a power socket in the kitchen
- Leisure: playing golf, obtaining and constructing new exercise equipment, holding books with both hands to read
- Walking to local shops, shopping in the supermarket
- Erecting and decorating the Christmas tree

'Getting down to business'

This section presents examples of Harry's occupational therapy sessions, linking relevant theory to practice. In all sessions, Harry was enabled to take control of the session and his recovery. Before performing occupations in therapy, I utilized adjunctive techniques (Pedretti, 1996) to normalize muscle tone in Harry's left upper limb and realign his subluxed shoulder. I also sought to promote generalization of learning by ensuring that Harry saw the links between skills and techniques used during different occupations.

Playing golf

After Harry had resumed independent driving in an adapted car, we arranged to meet at his local golf course. Harry was clearly happy to be at the golf course and this undoubtedly enhanced his sense of well-being. It seemed important to Harry that I also played golf, and this further reinforced our effective therapeutic relationship. As golf was unfamiliar to me, Harry explained the game and taught me how to hold a club; our roles had been reversed which Harry seemed to enjoy. Harry had difficulty holding a club with both hands and so I suggested that the correct grip could be facilitated by using a crepe bandage to keep his left hand on the club. This would allow joint movement because of its elasticity but would also help maintain his grip. From a distance, with the bandage roll tucked up his sleeve, the bandage looked like a glove. This was only a temporary solution as we needed to develop a strategy Harry could use independently. Harry's stamina and skill had deteriorated since his stroke and he was aware that he needed 'to start small and then grow', and so we confined ourselves to the putting green.

Watching Harry play golf was uplifting. He was emotionally and physically engaged with the game, paying attention and using smooth, fluid, normal movement patterns in a familar occupation that was rich with meaning. Harry's tendency to compare his current performance with his pre-stroke abilities entered our discussions, but he was still impressed with his abilities and elated to be on his beloved golf course. I used this as an opportunity to reinforce, yet again, the importance of completing meaningful and purposeful occupations to facilitate recovery from his stroke. This occupation reinforced three of Harry's priorities: holding a golf club in his left hand, reaching out to grip objects with his left hand (items from the boot of his car or on the table near the putting green, picking up a drink after the game) and bending down to pick up the golf balls with his right hand.

Making instant coffee

During this occupation, I facilitated movement in Harry's left upper limb so that he was able to complete making the coffee with the bilateral style he used prior to his stroke. To do this, I handled at the proximal key point of his shoulder joint and distal key point of his wrist and hand to facilitate the required movements. I asked Harry to concentrate on trying to complete the movements, talking himself through the sequence. It was vital that Harry actively participated in these movements and did not passively receive them. The aim was to help Harry complete the coffee making with his usual occupational style.

While making the coffee we shared stories about coffee drinking whilst on holidays and how I prefer brewed coffee to instant. This prompted Harry to remember that he had also enjoyed 'real coffee' prior to his stroke, but had changed to instant coffee because it seemed easier. It was touching to note that in subsequent sessions Harry made 'real coffee'. This session seemed to help cement our therapeutic relationship through shared meaning (Jackson, 1998). It also linked to a significant priority, reaching out with his left hand. He was able to use active elbow extension and needed considerable facilitation to maintain a grip on objects and to reach up into wall cupboards.

Mowing the lawn

Harry kept the lawn mower in his garage and needed to unlock and negotiate the side door to enter the garage in a narrow gap between the house and garage. I was interested to see if he would automatically implement the strategies we had used in other sessions for postural alignment. It was rewarding to see this generalization occur. Harry also decided to open the main garage door to exit with the lawn mower since this would be closer to the lawn. This showed effective problem-solving ability, a skill he had prior to his stroke and exhibited in many of our therapy sessions. Incorporating problem solving in therapy is an effective way to promote generalization (Birnboim, 1995; Brockman-Rubio, 1998; Sabari, 1998; Toglia, 1998; Hochstenbach & Mulder, 1999).

Harry effectively manoeuvred the lawn mower out of the garage and onto the lawn. He demonstrated how it worked so that I would be able to assist him. The mower was electrically powered and he demonstrated good safety awareness with the electric cable and circuit breaker. Pushing the mower required bilateral symmetrical positions of the upper limb joints. Harry could actively generate elbow extension and sufficient shoulder joint flexion, but I needed to facilitate left wrist extension so that Harry could maintain his grip on the handle and the start lever. As Harry walked up and down the small lawn, pushing the mower, I walked alongside him to facilitate left wrist extension and finger flexion. After ten minutes, Harry was able to maintain finger flexion independently but needed intermittent help with wrist extension. He actively negotiated obstacles such as small trees, a line of hedging and shrubs and even walked backwards, pulling the mower. This was something he had previously noted as difficult but had automatically done in the context of a familiar occupation. This lawn mowing session took 40 minutes in total, including setting up, emptying grass into the bin and putting away the mower. Throughout the session Harry maintained focus on the occupation, chatted about what he was doing and expressed satisfaction with his performance. This was the first time he had mowed the lawn since his stroke, and although he reported feeling fatigued, it was a 'good fatigue'.

Completing this occupation attended to two of Harry's priorities. Bending down to pick something up was achieved in plugging the mower into the extension lead, lifting the grass cutting box out of the mower, bending to reach for the low handle on the main garage door and bending to move the electric lead from the path of the mower. After two mowing sessions, Harry reported feeling so confident that he mowed independently, something he had previously thought too difficult.

Constructing exercise equipment

Harry had become bored with his limited repertoire of exercise equipment. He told me that he had ordered a folding bench with leg curl and knee extender. Once again, Harry was my teacher with another of his pastimes with which I was unfamiliar. He was gleeful as he relished another opportunity to share his knowledge. In the session the previous week I encouraged Harry to reflect on what he might find easy and difficult with this complex occupation. This strategy is part of the multicontext therapy approach, in particular metacognitive training (Toglia, 1991; Birnboim, 1995; Katz & Hartman-Maeir, 1997; Toglia, 1998). I asked him to make sure he had relevant tools ready and encouraged Harry to initiate and plan his use of time, something he often found difficult.

On the day, Harry was already in his garage when I arrived and he showed me part of the main framework that he had managed to assemble by himself. He had not managed to tighten bolts but had loosely located some of these, demonstrating his problem-solving skills, ability to follow written instructions and an awareness of his limitations. He also reported that his self-esteem had been boosted because he had managed to start the assembly process alone and related the skills needed to his previous employment. Harry took the lead in requesting my assistance when necessary. From our previous story sharing, he knew that I was familiar with tools and DIY and this enhanced his enthusiasm for the project. He recalled previous techniques I had used to facilitate movement in his upper limb and how he needed to use two hands to tighten bolts to keep the frame stable.

Using facilitation techniques to enable Harry to hold a spanner in his left hand, he was able to tighten bolts with ratchets in his right hand. He used a combination of bending whilst standing and kneeling to reach the bolts, which he found tiring. After 30 minutes, he requested that I kept bolts stable with the spanner whilst he tightened them. I thought that this might lead to some irritation but Harry remained content and focused. We worked in the garage for an hour and aimed to complete the project in the next session.

When I arrived for the next session, he had completed some more of the structure independently but had located two sections incorrectly. Harry was trying to understand why he could not complete the next stage. I drew his attention to the instruction sheets to see if he could spot his error. He found this very difficult and became quite frustrated. The complexity of the project had illustrated Harry's early therapy difficulties with visual motor processing. They were not totally resolved, but for his regular occupations they were not problematic. Harry and I talked about why he was having difficulty, but that he should not be too hard on himself as the task he was completing was very complex. Once I had pointed out the error Harry proceeded to solve the problem by using the diagram on the instructions. I felt it was important for his self-esteem that I did not explain what to do next, and his dissatisfaction with himself seemed temporary. He proceeded enthusiastically to demonstrate the use of the equipment by the end of the session.

Completing the construction of the exercise equipment contributed to Harry's identity as a fit man. It provided an opportunity for Harry to imagine a future through felt meanings and future images (Fleming & Mattingly, 1994; Jackson, 1998). This occupation also attended to some of Harry's priorities: reaching with his left hand and bending to pick up an object with his right hand.

11.3.4 Evaluating intervention

Harry was discharged from the community stroke service 18 months after his stroke. He was able to participate in many occupations that were important to him, contributing to his sense of identity and increasing his home based roles. He still missed his job as an engineer and the camaraderie at work. His high personal standards and difficulty in quickly moving his left upper limb resulted in a unilateral approach to some occupations, but overall he continued to persist in using his left side. The emotional consequences were still present but less problematic. He remained introspective and inclined to social isolation, partly due to the temporary loss of his driving licence following a minor seizure. Importantly, Harry was unable to get to the golf course independently but was looking forward to this in the near future. He was awaiting the manufacture of a specialized glove to help maintain the grip of his left hand on the golf club.

In considering Harry's five priorities, only one did not show significant progress: reaching for an object and gripping it with his left hand. Hypertonia in digit and wrist flexor muscles continued to influence his independence and sense of control, but he compensated for this difficulty by using his right hand. The NEADL (Nouri & Lincoln, 1987) was also completed again and showed that there were very few occupations that he either could not do or, more commonly, did not wish to do. Harry verbally reported his satisfaction with occupational therapy and wanted this to continue. Unfortunately, this was not possible due to restrictions placed on the service.

11.4 Conclusion

The purpose of this chapter was to demonstrate the importance of collaborating with clients on their journey through therapy. Occupational therapists use their own, and clients', stories to forge a therapeutic relationship. It is crucial to include meaning and relevance when constructing the therapy plan, using occupations to work towards shared goals and visions for the future; this is occupational therapy.

References

Ances, B.M. & D'Esposito, M. (2000). Neuroimaging of recovery of function after stroke: implications for rehabilitation. *Neurorehabilitation and Neural Repair, 14*, 171–179.

Bach-y-Rita, P. (2001). Theoretical and practical considerations in the restoration of function after stroke. *Topics in Stroke Rehabilitation, 8* (3), 1–15.

Birnboim, S. (1995). A metacognitive approach to cognitive rehabilitation. *British Journal of Occupational Therapy, 58* (2), 61–64.

Brockman-Rubio, K. (1998). Treatment of neurobehavioural deficits. In: G. Gillen & A. Burkhardt (Eds), *Stroke Rehabilitation. A Function Based Approach* (pp. 334–352). St Louis: Mosby.

Chollet, F., Di Piero, V., Wise, R.J.S., Brooks, D.J., Dolan, R.J. & Frackowiak, R.S.J. (1991). The functional anatomy of motor recovery after stroke in humans: a study with PET. *Annals of Neurology, 29* (1), 63–71.

Cramer, S.C., Nelles, G., Schaecter, J.D., Kaplan, J.D., Finklestein, S.P. & Rosen, B.R. (2001). A functional MRI study of three motor tasks in the evaluation of stroke recovery. *Neurorehabilitation and Neural Repair, 15* (1), 1–8.

Dean, C.M. & Shepherd, R.B. (1997). Task related training improves performance of seated reaching tasks after stroke. A RCT. *Stroke, 28,* 722–728.

Department of Health (2001). *The National Service Framework for Older People.* London: Department of Health.

Dolecheck, J.R. & Schkade, J.K. (1999). The extent dynamic standing endurance is affected when CVA subjects perform personally meaningful activities rather than non-meaningful tasks. *Occupational Therapy Journal of Research, 19* (1), 40–54.

Fisher, A.G. (1998). Uniting practice and theory in an occupational framework. *American Journal of Occupational Therapy, 52* (7), 509–521.

Fisher, B.E. & Sullivan, K.J. (2001). Activity-dependent factors affecting post-stroke functional outcomes. *Topics in Stroke Rehabilitation, 8* (3), 31–44.

Fleming, M. & Mattingly, C. (1994). Giving language to practice. In: C. Mattingly & M. Fleming (Eds), *Clinical Reasoning: Forms of Enquiry in a Therapeutic Practice.* Philadelphia: Lippincott.

Forsberg-Warleby, G. & Moller, A. (1996). Models of adaptation – an adaptation process after stroke analysed from different theoretical perspectives of adaptation. *Scandinavian Journal of Occupational Therapy, 3,* 114–122.

Giuffrida, C.G. (1998). Motor learning: an emerging frame of reference for occupational therapy. In: M.E. Neistadt & E.B. Crepeau (Eds), *Willard and Spackman's Occupational Therapy* (pp. 421–427). Philadelphia: Lippincott.

Goldman, S. & Plum, F. (1997). Compensatory regeneration of the damaged adult human brain: neuroplasticity in a clinical perspective. *Brain Plasticity, Advances in Neurology, 73,* 99–107.

Golledge, J. (1998). Distinguishing between occupation, purposeful activity and activity. Part 1: review and explanation. *British Journal of Occupational Therapy, 61* (3), 100–105.

Head, J. & Patterson, V. (1997). Performance context and its role in treatment planning. *American Journal of Occupational Therapy, 51* (6), 453–457.

Heddings, A.A., Friel, K.M., Plantz, E.J., Barbay, S. & Nudo, R.J. (2000). Factors contributing to motor impairment and recovery after stroke. *Neurorehabilitation and Neural Repair, 14* (4), 301–310.

Hochstenbach, J. & Mulder, T. (1999). Neuropsychology and the relearning of motor skills following stroke. *International Journal of Rehabilitation Research, 22,* 11–19.

Hocking, C. (2001). Implementing occupation based assessment. *American Journal of Occupational Therapy, 55* (4), 463–469.

Jackson, J. (1998). The value of occupation as the core of treatment: Sandy's experience. *American Journal of Occupational Therapy, 52* (6), 466–473.

Johannsson, B.B. (2000). Brain plasticity and stroke rehabilitation. *Stroke, 31,* 223–230.

Johnson, J.A. (1996). Occupational science and occupational therapy: an emphasis on meaning. In: R. Zemke & F. Clark (Eds), *Occupational Science. The Evolving Discipline* (pp. 393–397). Philadelphia: F.A. Davis.

Katz, N. & Hartman-Maeir, A. (1997). Occupational performance and metacognition. *Canadian Journal of Occupational Therapy, 64*, 53–62.

Lee, S.S., Powell, N.J. & Esdaile, S. (2001). A functional model of cognitive rehabilitation in occupational therapy. *Canadian Journal of Occupational Therapy, 68* (1), 41–50.

Lennon, S., Baxter, D. & Ashburn, A. (2001). Physiotherapy based on the Bobath concept in stroke rehabilitation: a survey within the UK. *Disability and Rehabilitation, 23* (6), 254–262.

Leonard, C.T. (1998). *The Neuroscience of Human Movement*. St Louis: Mosby.

Levin, H. & Grafman, J. (Eds) (2000). *Neuroplasticity and Reorganization of Function after Brain Injury*. New York: Oxford University Press.

Liepert, J., Bauder, H., Miltner, W.H.R., Taub, E. & Weiller, C. (2000). Treatment induced cortical reorganization after stroke in humans. *Stroke, 31*, 1210–1216.

Ma, H., Trombly, C.A. & Robinson-Podolski, C. (1999). The effect of context on skill acquisition and transfer. *American Journal of Occupational Therapy, 53* (2), 138–144.

Mahoney, S.I. & Barthel, D.W. (1965). Functional Evaluation – Barthel Index. *Maryland State Medical Journal, 14*, 61–65.

Mathiowetz, V. & Bass Haugen, J. (1994). Motor behaviour research: implications for therapeutic approaches to CNS dysfunction. *American Journal of Occupational Therapy, 48* (8), 733–745.

Neistadt, M.E. (1998). Overview of treatment. In: M.E. Neistadt & E.B. Crepeau (Eds), *Willard and Spackman's Occupational Therapy* (pp. 315–322). Philadelphia: Lippincott.

Nelson, D.L., Konosky, K., Fleharty, K., Webb, R., Newer, K., Hazboun, V.P., Fontane, C. & Licht, B.C. (1996). The effects of an occupationally embedded exercise on bilaterally assisted supination in persons with hemiplegia. *American Journal of Occupational Therapy, 50* (8), 639–646.

Nouri, F.M. & Lincoln, N.B. (1987). An extended activities of daily living scale for stroke patients. *Clinical Rehabilitation, 1*, 301–305.

Panturin, E. (2001). The Bobath concept. (Letter) *Clinical Rehabilitation, 15*, 111.

Pedretti, L.W. (1996). Occupational performance: a model for practice in physical dysfunction. In: L.W. Pedretti (Ed.), *Occupational Therapy. Practice Skills for Physical Dysfunction* (pp. 3–12). St Louis: Mosby.

Rice, M.S., Alaimo, A.J. & Cook, J.A. (1999). Movement dynamics and occupational embeddedness in a grasping and placing task. *Occupational Therapy International, 6* (4), 298–310.

Rudd, A., Goldacre, M., Amess, M., Fletcher, J., Wilkinson, E., Mason, A., Fairfield, G., Eastwood, A., Cleary, R. & Coles, J. (1999). *Health Outcome Indicators: Stroke. Report of a working group to the Department of Health*. Oxford: National Centre for Health Outcomes Development.

Sabari, J.S. (1998). Application of learning and environmental strategies to activity based treatment. In: G. Gillen & A. Burkhardt (Eds), *Stroke Rehabilitation. A Function Based Approach* (pp. 31–46). St Louis: Mosby.

Selzer, M.E. (2000). Neural plasticity and repair in rehabilitation. *Neurorehabilitation and Neural Repair, 14* (4), 245–249.

Shumway-Cook, A. & Woollacott, M.H. (2001). *Motor Control: Theory and Practical Applications* (2nd edn). Philadelphia: Lippincott Williams and Wilkins.

Stephen, A. & Rafferty, J. (Eds) (1994). *Health Care Needs Assessment*. Oxford: Radcliffe Medical Press.

Toglia, J.P. (1991). Generalization of treatment: a multicontext approach. *American Journal of Occupational Therapy*, 45 (6), 505–515.

Toglia, J.P. (1998). A dynamic interactional model to cognitive rehabilitation. In: N. Katz (Ed.), *Cognition and Occupation in Rehabilitation*. Bethesda: American Occupational Therapy Association.

Unsworth, C.A. & Cunningham, D.T. (2002). Examining the evidence base for occupational therapy with clients following stroke. *British Journal of Occupational Therapy*, 65 (1), 21–29.

Van Vliet, P., Sheridan, M., Kerwin, D.G. & Fentem, P. (1995). The influence of functional goals on the kinematics of reaching following stroke. *Neurology Report*, 19 (1), 11–16.

Whiting, S., Lincoln, N., Bhavnani, G. & Cockburn, J. (1985). *Rivermead Perceptual Assessment Battery*. Windsor: NFER Nelson.

Wilcock, A. (1998). *An Occupational Perspective of Health*. Thorofare: Slack.

Wilson, B., Cockburn, J. & Halligan, P. (1987). *Behavioural Inattention Test*. Bury St. Edmonds: Thames Valley Testing Company.

Wolf, C., Rudd, A. & Beech, R. (1996). *Stroke Services and Research. An Overview with Recommendations for Future Research*. London: Stroke Association.

Wu, C., Trombly, C.A., Lin, K. & Tickle-Degnen, L. (1998). Effects of object affordances on reaching performance in persons with and without CVA. *American Journal of Occupational Therapy*, 52 (6), 447–456.

Yerxa, E.J. (1998). Occupation: a keystone of a curriculum for a self defined profession. *American Journal of Occupational Therapy*, 52 (5), 365–372.

Chapter 12
Occupational Science: The Forensic Challenge

Jane Cronin-Davis, Amanda Lang and Matthew Molineux[1]

12.1 Introduction

Although there is evidence to suggest that occupation is important in achieving and maintaining mental health, there is little indication that occupational therapists use occupation as the primary means of their intervention (Legault & Rebeiro, 2001). Despite this, the therapeutic use of occupation in different settings has been outlined. The practice areas addressed in the literature include prisons and mainstream mental health services (Townsend, 1997; Lambert, 1998; Rebeiro *et al.*, 2001). There is, however, a dearth of evidence relating to forensic psychiatry.

This chapter seeks to suggest how occupational science can be used to guide occupational therapy assessment and treatment of patients in forensic psychiatry settings. It is borne out of a continuing professional development initiative at Stockton Hall Hospital, a private medium secure hospital in York, United Kingdom. This initiative was driven by the occupational therapy team's desire to reflect and understand clinical practice in an innovative way. The chapter will begin with a brief overview of occupational therapy in forensic psychiatry, followed by a discussion of how occupational science can inform this developing area of clinical practice. A case study will then be outlined to show how occupational risk factors relate to the assessment and treatment of patients in forensic settings.

12.2 Overview

Forensic psychiatry is the interface between mental health services and the criminal justice system. As such, it is concerned with the assessment and treatment of individuals who have acute or chronic mental health difficulties, a

[1] The work carried out by the occupational therapists at Stockton Hall Hospital, York, has underpinned much of the material contained in this chapter. Grateful thanks go to Flippa Watkeys, Ruth Longworth-Zuercher, Leanne Jones, Louisa Littler, Rachel Young, Naomi Smith, Neil Morgan and Ian Davey.

learning disability, personality disorder, problems with substance abuse, or a combination of these. In addition, most of the patients in forensic services have committed, or been charged with, a criminal offence. Some individuals may be admitted to forensic services from general mental health units because their behaviour has been unmanageable (e.g. persistent absconding or posing a danger to themselves or others) and thus require increased levels of security. The forensic population is predominantly white, single men, from low socio-economic groups who have generally not worked prior to admission (Thompson *et al.*, 1997). For many patients, their occupational abilities, choices and opportunities have often been eroded due to the effects of long-term institutionalization. Some patients may have had limited opportunities to develop a sense of themselves as competent occupational beings due to the impact of the contexts in which they grew up and lived.

Forensic services span many sectors including prisons, secure hospitals and the community, and patients can often transfer between these different settings and levels of security depending on assessed risk. The ultimate goal of forensic services is usually for the patient to reintegrate back into the community with a comprehensive care and treatment programme which addresses ongoing needs and risk management.

Occupational therapy was recognized by the inquiry into the provision of services for forensic psychiatry clients as a vital component of the rehabilitation process within forensic settings (Reed, 1992). Since then, there has been a growth in the number of occupational therapists working in this varied, challenging and demanding clinical area, and the specific contribution of the profession has been recognized (Chacksfield, 1997; Flood, 1997; Baker & McKay, 2001). The conceptualization of humans as occupational beings is a particularly valuable perspective in this setting. In forensic services it is important to remember that rehabilitation should not be limited to teaching patients skills for domestic tasks (Blackburn, 1996). Flannigan (1996) suggested that the focus of occupational therapy in forensic psychiatry is to address the loss of autonomy and to empower the patient to take responsibility.

It is also important to acknowledge that the nature of secure environments can limit patients' access to a diverse range of occupations, which might be available to them in other settings. In addition, patients may have their own inherent risks: propensity for violence, self-injurious behaviour, unpredictability, impulsivity, attempts to abscond or escape, sexual aggression, arson, illicit substance abuse and treatment resistive psychosis. Although there is a continuing debate as to whether people with schizophrenia do have a higher propensity for violence than others with an Axis 1 diagnosis, Prins (1999, p. 46) suggested that apart from 'severe personality disorder, schizophrenic illnesses seem to have the strongest relationship to the commission of serious violence'. These issues mean that all stages of occupational therapy intervention can be hindered by characteristics of the patients and/or the forensic environment.

Occupational science provides a framework which enables the occupational therapist to understand the complexities of patients in a forensic setting. It acknowledges the wider issues and external influences of a patient's circumstances and psychopathology, and provides a vehicle for the comprehensive exploration of risk factors. The unique challenges that face occupational therapists working in this area are twofold: the first is the ever present risk posed by patients, and second is the need to be resourceful and creative in facilitating occupational engagement relevant to these risks. Occupational therapists can use the framework provided by occupational science to organize and inform clinical interventions from admission to eventual discharge.

12.3   An approach to practice informed by occupational science

For occupational therapy to be maximally effective within a forensic setting, we suggest that occupational therapists must adopt a view of their clients as occupational beings, or to use the phrase coined by Yerxa (2000, p. 197) as *homo occupacio*:

> 'a self-organizing system who responds to specific environmental challenges, with occupation, creating an adaptive response. Successful self-organization creates skill, which will be available in the face of new, unknown challenges.'

The perspective proposed here requires that occupational therapy assessment must establish the causes of occupational dysfunction, in particular to identify the occupational risk factors impacting on the individual. These risk factors include performance deficits, occupational disruption, occupational imbalance, occupational deprivation, occupational alienation, or a combination of these. Once the cause of occupational dysfunction has been established, occupational therapy treatment involves improving occupational function through occupational enrichment: 'the deliberate manipulation of environments to facilitate and support engagement in a range of occupations congruent with those the individual might normally perform' (Molineux & Whiteford, 1999, p. 127). Occupational enrichment can be both the process and outcome of treatment, that is, methods can be implemented to address the occupational risk factors, but also that the aim of occupational therapy might be an occupationally enriched environment. The proposed framework is presented in Figure 12.1 and its elements are outlined briefly below.

12.3.1   Occupational risk factors

Performance deficits are those which impact on the individual at the level of occupational performance components (American Occupational Therapy Association, 1994), such as sensorimotor, cognitive or psychosocial elements of occupational performance. Deficits in these areas are likely to be associated with the psychiatric condition of the individual, such as hallucinations or delusions, or concomitant physical difficulties such as asthma, arthritis or a hand injury.

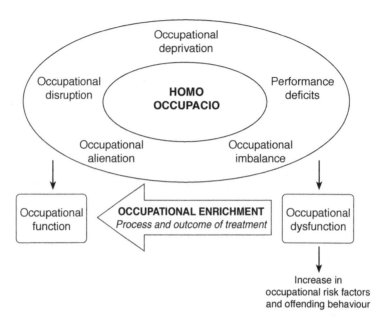

Figure 12.1 Conceptualizing the occupational therapy process and occupational risk factors in forensic psychiatry. (Developed from original work by Stockton Hall Hospital Occupational Therapy Service.)

Occupational disruption has been proposed in the literature to refer to the transient or temporary inability to engage in occupations due to life events, environmental changes or acute illness or injury (Whiteford, 2000). For individuals within forensic settings these might include living away from family and friends, living in a secure environment and moving between different institutions.

Occupational deprivation has been defined as 'the deprivation of occupational choice and diversity due to circumstances beyond the control of the individual' (Wilcock, 1998, p. 257). This is distinct from occupational disruption, as deprivation occurs over an extended period of time and so is not transient or temporary (Whiteford, 1997). Occupational deprivation may have been a long-standing issue for some clients due to impoverished lives during childhood or in the time leading up to contact with forensic services. The very nature of the forensic environment also places people at risk of occupational deprivation, given that it is often necessary to restrict patient access to the wider community or certain occupations that require tools or materials which some may use against themselves or others. Whiteford (1997) has suggested, based on her study of occupational deprivation in a maximum security prison in New Zealand, that rigid no-tool policies contributed to inmates' reduced capacity to initiate and engage in occupations. In addition, the impoverished and isolated environmental conditions lead to the lack of opportunities for orientation in time and social interaction through occupations.

Occupational alienation refers to the subjective experiences of 'isolation, powerlessness, frustration, loss of control, estrangement from society or self' which results from engagement in occupations which fail to satisfy the inner needs of the individual (Wilcock, 1998, p. 257). The very limited opportunities for choice available to patients in some forensic settings may lead to occupational alienation. So too, might the sense of separation from wider society while being held in secure units away from family, friends, their community and preferred social networks.

Finally, *occupational imbalance* refers to the loss of a balance of engagement in occupations which leads to well-being, and might include balance between physical, mental and social occupations; between chosen and obligatory occupations; or between doing and being (Wilcock, 1998). For many of the reasons which have already been outlined in the preceding paragraphs, patients may not be able to experience a balance of health-giving occupations.

Although the focus of this chapter is forensic psychiatry, all individuals could be seen as being exposed to all of the occupational risk factors just described. Despite the presence of these risk factors, many individuals are able to achieve occupational functioning and live a life that is occupationally enriched, balanced and contributes to a sense of well-being. However, due to their life history, in addition to their mental health difficulties, patients in forensic settings are likely to have experienced occupational risk factors to such a degree that they have been unable to achieve or maintain a state of occupational functioning. Furthermore, the very nature of secure environments can further compound the impact of any occupational risk factors. It is not suggested that all patients in forensic settings will experience all of the occupational risk factors identified here, but it is proposed that at least some are likely to be present for many patients.

12.3.2 Occupational therapy treatment

Occupational therapy treatment is likely to involve addressing, as much as is possible, the occupational risk factors which are resulting in occupational dysfunction. This might include more traditional interventions to address performance deficits, such as time management or social skills training. It might also include occupational enrichment strategies. These may encompass methods such as providing opportunities for patients to engage in a range of occupations either alone or within groups. It may also involve addressing wider systemic issues within forensic services or institutions, such as policies on access to the community, employment programmes and family contact opportunities. While it is the ultimate aim of occupational therapy to enable patients to experience occupational enrichment and achieve occupational functioning, it can be hugely challenging within secure environments, and so the skills of occupational therapists in devising treatment programmes with, and for, their clients will require a creative and versatile skill base.

Within the forensic environment, occupational enrichment may be difficult to achieve due to patients' often distorted perceptions of meaningful occupations. Patients may also have unrealistic views of their future lives due to a lack of insight into their mental health needs and criminal behaviour. The difficulties these issues cause for patients are also felt by occupational therapists as they struggle to ensure that occupations used in therapy are relevant to the patient. All these factors must be incorporated into the decision making processes of occupational therapists as they seek to construct experiences which are not only meaningful for clients, but also consistent with socio-cultural values and expectations. Difficult as this may be, it is crucial in order to engage the patient in therapy and maximize the chances of therapy being successful (Mattingly, 1991). For example, how do occupational therapists substitute previously lucrative, and in some ways adaptive, occupations such as shoplifting, sexual offences, stalking, football hooliganism, and instrumental aggression, for more socially accepted occupations?

The contradiction inherent in this approach is that the very intervention offered may itself cause occupational disruption and so further contribute, hopefully only temporarily, to a state of occupational dysfunction. The authors propose that the occupational therapy process can move patients from a state of occupational dysfunction to occupational functioning through occupational enrichment. Identifying a patient's goals of therapy help to empower the patient, facilitate engagement in the therapeutic process and increase a patient's feelings of self-worth. The study by Mee and Sumsion (2001) suggests that engagement in purposeful occupation stimulates intrinsic motivation, builds competence and helps develop self-identity. In this way patients learn to view their world more positively and experience a greater degree of functioning in areas such as productivity, performance and motivation.

12.4   Case study: John

John was a 29 year-old man who had been referred from the prison service to a medium security forensic unit as he was considered a high risk for escape, violence against others and taking a hostage. Prior to transfer to the forensic unit's assessment ward, John had spent two months on the prison hospital wing receiving treatment for florid psychosis which involved a complex delusional system, including a belief that a male doctor could read his mind and was monitoring both his thoughts and actions. His symptoms were not responding to antipsychotic medication and so referral to the forensic unit was made in the hope of establishing his potential longer-term treatment needs. John had been in the prison system for approximately five years prior to his transfer. He had been convicted of perverting the course of justice and the murder, with four acquaintances, of a young girl. John received a mandatory life sentence.

Soon after his admission to the assessment unit John was referred for an occupational therapy assessment in order to establish a baseline of his occupational function/dysfunction, with a view to him being involved in occupational therapy intervention. Within two days of admission the occupational therapist interviewed John and explained the occupational therapy assessment process which included, in John's case, the following assessments: Occupational

Performance History Interview, version II (Kielhofner *et al.*, 1998); Assessment of Communication and Interaction Skills (Forsyth *et al.*, 1998); Occupational Therapy Task Observation Scale (Margolis, 1996); Occupational Self Assessment (Baron *et al.*, 1999); informal interviews; review of psychiatric and prison reports; ward based observations; and assessment of domestic and self-care occupations. Many of the individual sessions involved cooking, due to John's stated preference for this particular occupation as an assessment medium. The full assessment process took place over three months, and although lengthy and time consuming it proved valuable in understanding John and his occupational performance needs; and enabled negotiation of a proposed occupational therapy treatment programme aimed at enriching his immediate environment.

12.4.1   Occupational history

John's childhood was characterized by disruption. His father was unemployed and regularly beat his wife, John and his six siblings. John was the eldest son in the family and so felt responsible for looking after his mother and the other children, and this continued into adulthood. Although John's academic achievements were poor he felt that he had adequate literacy and numeracy skills. Prior to being sentenced, John was earning a good income for a number of years as a professional thief. He employed four other people and the 'team' would shoplift to order. John had never held any legal employment. He lived with his wife, who did not work, and their four children. John also had two other children who were the result of long-term extramarital relationships. He stated that he had many acquaintances but no real friends, and described himself as a loner.

   When asked about hobbies or interests, John reported engaging in illicit drug use and visiting nightclubs. He had prior convictions for drug related driving and acquisitive offences, and had also been charged with grievous bodily harm. During his time in custody, John was frequently moved between prisons which made it difficult to feel settled or to truly acclimatize to his surroundings. He was able to identify some occupations which he enjoyed: cooking meals for fellow prisoners, attending the gym on a regular basis and working with the prison garden team.

12.4.2   Occupational performance and occupational risk factors

John was independent in most aspects of self-care and so washed and dressed independently. Occasionally, when his mental state deteriorated, he required prompting from the nursing staff to shower. In terms of productivity occupations, John kept his room tidy and laundered his own clothes. During cooking sessions John often asked for guidance and sought reassurance from the occupational therapist, despite his high level of competence. The only leisure occupation John was able to identify was attending the prison gym twice each day. From the time of admission to the forensic unit, however, John chose not to continue this leisure pursuit, citing interference from the male doctor in his delusion as the reason.

Prior to the onset of his illness, whilst in prison, John was able to manage his occupational performance so that he engaged in a range of occupations which he found stimulating and rewarding. During the assessment period, John spent the majority of his time in his hospital room and did not engage in any activities unless these were initiated by and performed in conjunction with staff.

Occupational disruption

John had experienced occupational disruptions throughout his life. As a child his home environment was violent and he did not attend school regularly. Whilst in prison, he was frequently moved from one institution to another. Initially, John did not respond well to his transfer from prison to the hospital, as he lacked insight into the need for assessment and treatment of his mental health difficulties.

Occupational deprivation

John had very limited access to occupations within the hospital due to his legal detention under the Mental Health Act 1983. He was a restricted patient under Section 47/49 of the Act and so could not leave the hospital ward or exercise compound without prior permission from the Home Office. In addition, his delusional belief that he was being observed and controlled by a male doctor often meant that he would refuse to take part in the occupations offered to him for fear that he would not perform to what he perceived to be his usual high standards.

Occupational alienation

John had always felt that he was different from others and during the assessment process he appeared very socially anxious and demonstrated low self-esteem. During the initial stages of his assessment period John did not associate with the other patients on the ward and would only interact with staff. He refused to accept the need for admission to a hospital or that he had mental health problems. His long-term incarceration meant that he lost a sense of connection with his usual community, and he had infrequent contact with family members. John did not speak to the mother of his children and had no awareness of where they lived.

Occupational imbalance

In the hospital setting, when not engaged in a staff-initiated activity, John spent much of his day isolated in his room. Prior to the onset of his mental health problems John kept himself busy, either working in the prison gardens or kitchens, or participating in gym activities. Before his prison sentence, John structured his day conducting his criminal activities, using illicit substances and going to nightclubs. He was concerned about his lack of progress in the prison system, and had major worries about his long-term employment options. John realized that these would now be limited due to his criminal convictions.

12.4.3   Intervention

A multidisciplinary treatment intervention programme was formulated and included ongoing assessment and monitoring of John's mental state, stabilization of his mental state by the prescription and administration of antipsychotic medication, cognitive behavioural therapy aimed at reducing the frequency and intensity of delusional ideation and re-establishing contact with family members. The occupational therapy programme aimed to promote occupational enrichment and maintain occupational performance skills.

An initial occupational therapy treatment plan was formulated to provide John with opportunities for occupational engagement. The aims of this were:

- To promote and maintain a high level of occupational performance.
- To acknowledge and explore self-esteem issues in order to enable John to participate in relevant occupations.
- To assist John to overcome his social anxiety using an occupation based desensitization programme.
- To acknowledge and discuss negative symptomology and how this impacted on John's initiation of and engagement in occupations.
- To assess and monitor ongoing occupational risk factors.

The concept of occupational enrichment was utilized to grade and adapt both the treatment plan and clinical environment by measured exposure to gardening and cookery sessions, which were initially with the ward-based occupational therapist. These were occupations specifically chosen with John as they were relevant and meaningful to him. After a period of three months, and following the desensitization programme, John commenced work with technical instructors in different environments within the hospital setting, continuing with his chosen occupations. In addition, John received ongoing individual sessions with the ward-based occupational therapist, which incorporated continued mental health assessment and monitoring, psychosocial education, and monitoring of occupational performance.

It was important that John's occupational therapy assessment and subsequent treatment programme were occupationally based. Use of the occupations chosen by John meant that he was able to engage in occupational therapy without feeling pressured or exposed. His chosen occupations were readily available within the occupational therapy service and were easily managed in relation to John's potential to abscond and become violent. Using occupations in this way meant that John's occupational therapy was a process of *doing* which enabled discussion and collaboration between the occupational therapist and John.

Regular evaluation took place in discussion with John and outcome measures, such as the Assessment of Communication and Interactions Skills and the Occupational Therapy Task Observation Scale, were used to monitor his progress. The outcome of occupational therapy intervention was that a high level of functional performance continued despite severe fluctuations in John's mental state. He began to demonstrate some initial insight into his delusions, albeit with some residual beliefs. With the reduction in assessed risk factors John was able to work outside in secure compound areas. During his individual sessions John began to explore occupational alternatives beyond that of a 'lifer', after release from prison. A recommendation was made for John to transfer to a unit with lower security.

12.5 Conclusion

Occupational therapists are undoubtedly a recognizable force within the forensic arena. It is an ever-growing discipline, which has a specific contribution to the assessment, treatment and rehabilitation of this patient group. It is imperative that this growth continues so that the impact of aspects of forensic psychiatry services on occupational therapy interventions can be better understood. This growth is in parallel with the development of the profession as a more robust field. Occupational science is crucial to this clinical area as it provides a framework for occupational therapists to understand patients with complex pathologies and consequently enhance clinical practice. It will assist our understanding of patients' occupational behaviours and how these have affected their criminogenic needs. One of the key skills of an occupational therapist is the ability to engage and motivate patients by using a diversity of occupations. Using this process and developing the necessary treatment interventions, occupational therapists can assist patients to address their occupational risk factors. Occupational therapists must ensure interventions not only recognize patients' forensic pathology, but they must be proactive in addressing how patients' criminal occupations impact on their lifestyle and well-being. This is the unique contribution of occupational therapy within this clinical speciality.

References

American Occupational Therapy Association (1994). Uniform terminology for occupational therapy. (3rd edn). *American Journal of Occupational Therapy*, 48 (11), 1047–1054.

Baker, S. & McKay, E. (2001). Occupational therapists' perspectives of the needs of women in medium secure units. *British Journal of Occupational Therapy*, 64 (9), 441–448.

Baron, K., Kielhofner, G., Goldhammer, V. & Wolenski, J. (1999). *Occupational Self Assessment*. Chicago: University of Illinois at Chicago.

Blackburn, R. (1996). Working with offenders. In: C. Hollin (Ed.) *Working with Offenders: Psychological Practice in Offender Rehabilitation* (p. 119–149). London: John Wiley.

Chacksfield, J. (1997). Forensic occupational therapy: is it a developing specialism? *British Journal of Therapy and Rehabilitation*, 4 (7), 371–374.

Flannigan, E. (1996). The occupational therapist. In: M. Cordess & C. Cox (Eds), *Forensic Psychotherapy*. London: Jessica Kingsley.

Flood, B. (1997). An introduction to occupational therapy in forensic psychiatry. *British Journal of Therapy and Rehabilitation*, 4 (7), 375–379.

Forsyth, K., Lai, J. & Kielhofner, G. (1998). *Assessment of Communication and Interaction Skills*. Chicago: University of Illinois at Chicago.

Kielhofner, G., Mallinson, T., Crawford, C., Nowak, M., Rigby, M., Henry, A. & Walens, D. (1998). *A User's Manual for the Occupational Performance History Interview.* Chicago: Model of Human Occupation Clearinghouse.

Lambert, R. (1998). Occupation and lifestyle: implications for mental health practice. *British Journal of Occupational Therapy, 61* (5), 193–197.

Legault, E. & Rebeiro, K. (2001). Occupation as a means to mental health: a single-case study. *American Journal of Occupational Therapy, 55* (1), 90–96.

Margolis, R.L. (1996). *Occupational Therapy Task Observation Scale.* Chicago: University of Illinois at Chicago.

Mattingly, C. (1991). The narrative nature of clinical reasoning. *American Journal of Occupational Therapy, 45* (11), 998–1005.

Mee, J. & Sumsion, T. (2001). Mental health clients confirm the motivating power of occupation. *British Journal of Occupational Therapy, 64* (3), 121–128.

Mental Health Act 1983. London: HMSO.

Molineux, M. & Whiteford, G. (1999). Prisons: from occupational deprivation to occupational enrichment. *Journal of Occupational Science, 6* (3), 124–130.

Prins, H. (1999). *Will They Do it Again?* London: Routledge.

Rebeiro, K., Day, D., Semeniuk, B., O'Brien, M. & Wilson, B. (2001). Northern initiative for social action: an occupation-based mental health programme. *American Journal of Occupational Therapy, 55* (5), 493–500.

Reed, J. (1992). *The Final Summary of the Committee into the Provision of Services for Mentally Disordered Offenders.* London: HMSO.

Thompson, L., Bogue, J., Humphreys, M., Owens, D. & Johnstone, E. (1997). State hospital survey: a description of psychiatric patients in conditions of special security in Scotland. *Journal of Forensic Psychiatry, 8* (2), 263–284.

Townsend, E. (1997). Occupation: potential for personal and social transformation. *Journal of Occupational Science: Australia, 4* (1), 18–26.

Whiteford, G. (1997). Occupational deprivation and incarceration. *Journal of Occupational Science: Australia, 4* (3), 126–130.

Whiteford, G. (2000). Occupational deprivation: global challenges in the new millennium. *British Journal of Occupational Therapy, 63* (5), 200–204.

Wilcock, A. (1998). *An Occupational Perspective of Health.* Thorofare: Slack.

Yerxa, E. (2000). Confessions of an occupational therapist who became a detective. *British Journal of Occupational Therapy, 63* (5), 192–199.

Section C
Future Possibilities

Chapter 13
Occupational Issues of Refugees

Gail Elizabeth Whiteford

13.1 Introduction

The last two decades have witnessed an unprecedented growth in the number of refugees globally. Whilst the reasons for this dramatic growth in numbers are complex, and include, for example, nation state conflicts and minority group persecution, the bald fact remains that this large number of people have needs which must be addressed. As reinforced by the United Nations High Commission on Refugees (UNHCR), all people have the right to seek asylum and find safe refuge in another state. Clearly the collective governments of countries around the world have a role to play in protecting and supporting this inalienable right.

Whilst the phenomenon of refugeeism is complex and multifaceted, this chapter considers the needs of refugees from an occupational perspective. Specifically, the objectives of this chapter are to:

- Provide historic, legal and demographic background on refugeeism.
- Consider the occupational issues and needs of refugees.
- Present some suggestions for occupationally focused action and interventions.
- Reflect on future roles and directions in this area.

Accordingly, the chapter's structure will reflect these objectives. The first section will provide the reader with some important knowledge of the phenomenon of refugeeism and asylum seeking around the globe. Given this background, the occupational issues and needs of refugees, will be presented in the second section and are based on both a review of current literature as well as on research currently being undertaken by the author. In the third section, suggestions for occupationally focused action, activism and intervention, based on the issues and needs identified in section two, are presented for reflection and consideration. The final section will forecast future trends with respect to refugees and the potential for occupationally focused strategies and interventions.

13.2   Overview: refugees and asylum seekers

13.2.1   Refugees and asylum seekers: differences and issues

The term refugee, as understood in the international community, comes from the 1951 United Nations convention on the status of refugees, which states:

> 'A refugee is a person who owing to a well founded fear of being persecuted for reasons of race, religion, nationality, membership of a particular social group or political opinion, is outside the country of his nationality and is unable or, owing to such fear, is unwilling to avail himself of the protection of that country.' (UNHCR, 2002a).

As is evident from this definition, people become refugees when they need to leave their country because of violence, persecution or threat thereof (Goodwin-Gill, 1996). Refugees are those people who migrate to other countries, usually through humanitarian or similar programmes and are accepted into that country through authorized channels. Once in their new country of resettlement, they have rights and privileges similar to other citizens. Criminals who have received a fair trial in their country of origin are not considered refugees, nor are soldiers or war criminals (UNHCR, 2002a).

Asylum seekers are different in status, at least initially, from refugees. They are people who, in fleeing from war, conflict, violence and/or persecution enter a country either in an authorized manner, for example with a student or visitor's visa and are then allowed to stay, or who enter in an unauthorized manner (Smith, 2001). In Australia, for example, asylum seekers have arrived in boats via Indonesia to escape regimes and conflicts in places such as Afghanistan and Iraq. Such people are currently held in detention centres whilst their applications for protection visas are processed by the Department of Immigration and Multicultural Affairs. It should be noted that policies of mandatory detention, such as those enacted in Australia, have been variously described as: the most draconian punishment known to most liberal democratic countries (Loff, 2002); representing direct violations of several international treaties on human rights (Sidoti, 2002); representing one of the most severe policies in a Western democratic country (McMaster, 2002); inhumane and unwarranted (Jupp, 2002); and ruinous to Australia's reputation internationally (McMaster, 2002). Additionally, mandatory detention has been identified as having serious negative health and psychological consequences (Silove & Steel, 1998; Sultan & O'Sullivan, 2001).

From these descriptions it is clear that the person or family group who are able to pursue legally sanctioned processes to gain refugee status, fare better in their country of resettlement, in terms of rights and recognition, than asylum seekers who enter illegally. Given that the number of asylum seekers is increasing, however, the question that is begged, is how asylum seekers are to be best treated with respect to health, welfare and occupational needs in the countries into which they arrive. Clearly, economic issues notwithstanding, policies and practices in this area require closer examination and development along humanitarian principles (Sidoti, 2002).

Internationally the number of refugees has grown in the last 20 years, with current global estimates being approximately 20 million (see Table 13.1). It should be noted that 'internally displaced persons', that is, those who may be fleeing conflict within their country temporarily but are not legally considered to be refugees, are not included in these figures, but are estimated to be approximately 20–25 million in number (UNHCR, 2002a).

Table 13.1   Estimates of persons whose concerns fall under the mandate of the UNHCR, 1 January 2002 (UNHCR, 2002a)

Region	Number
Asia	8 820 700
Europe	4 855 400
Africa	4 173 500
Northern America	1 086 800
Latin America and Caribbean	765 400
Oceania	81 300
Total	**19 783 100**

13.2.2   The role of the UNHCR

The UNHCR is mandated by a statute of the United Nations and was established on 14 December 1950, beginning work the following year. It currently has an active staff of approximately 5000 people in more than 120 countries. The role of the UNHCR (2002a) is to protect the rights of refugees worldwide and to ensure that everyone can exercise their right to seek asylum in another state and return home voluntarily.

Besides dealing with the immediate issues of refugees globally, the UNHCR also has a role in ensuring the creation of a new home and achievement of equal status in a refugee's country of resettlement. Interestingly, occupational participation is seen as central to this process, which is described as one in which a refugee is provided with 'the means of building a new life and a way to help him direct his thoughts and activities into constructive channels … a chance to participate fully in the vital endeavours where he is needed' (Schnyder, 1962, p. 3). That occupational participation (in its broadest sense, not just in the occupation of paid employment) is also an important means through which the effects of trauma, torture and refugeeism can be ameliorated is reinforced by Garner (2001). He comments on the fact that a recent UK study into the backgrounds of asylum seekers and refugees determined that this group were likely to be well educated and skilled. Accordingly, he encourages greater consideration of employment and community options for asylum seekers and refugees as a response to labour force shortages, as a means to reduce the negative impacts of refugeeism and to expedite the process of community integration in the host country.

13.2.3   The current issues

As is evident from the figures above, the sheer number of refugees worldwide is an issue in itself. Whilst countries such as the US, Germany, Canada, the UK and Australia have in the past been committed to substantial numbers of refugees through planned humanitarian intake programmes, there is evidence a growing lack of preparedness to maintain such a commitment in the face of global and regional increases (Jupp, 2002). For security reasons the number of people arriving in countries illegally to seek asylum is of particular concern to governments.

A significant issue that is only beginning to receive adequate attention in the international arena, is the welfare of women and children who are dis-proportionately represented in the overall refugee statistics. Women are victims of persecution, physical and sexual violence (Goodwin-Gill, 1996), which occurs for a number of complex and often intersecting reasons. Pittaway and Bartolomei (2002, p. 19) provide a powerful description of this scenario:

'Refugee women are actively discriminated against on the grounds of their ethnicity and their gender. In terms of racial discrimination they are often devalued or "othered" on the grounds of their race and this effectively removes any need by the aggressors to respect them by gender. This "others" them twice and makes them prime targets for systematic rape and sexual torture for the purpose of shaming the men of their communities ... they are raped by the military, by border guards and by the UN peacekeeping forces sent to protect them. Rape is the most common form of systematized torture used against women.'

Additionally, Williams (1990) contends that women often face violence from their own husbands and family members whilst in the destabilizing environment of the refugee camp. Whilst this is a situation that should be of grave and urgent concern, recognition of this has been relatively slow amongst organizations and government departments (Williams, 1990; Pittaway & Bartolomei, 2002). An international report on refugee women (UNHCR, 2002b, p. 1) reinforces this point and states categorically that:

'refugee women continue to be disproportionately affected by physical and sexual violence and abuse ... International laws, standards and policies on this issue abound: the problem is that they are inadequately implemented.'

In summary, refugees, whether male or female, adult or child, face a number of serious and potentially life-threatening concerns whether in their home country, in camps or in their country of resettlement. Whilst the issues of safety, adequate access to food and shelter and basic amenities are immediate and pressing, the need to re-engage in meaningful occupations, to re-establish familiar routines and to connect with others, is also important, though often unacknowledged in the planning and delivery of aid and assistance. How these needs can be addressed is the focus of the next section.

13.3   Establishing client needs

Whilst the literature collectively highlights some of the occupational and other issues of refugees en masse, establishing the needs of such a group of people is difficult for a number of reasons. First, the very nature of refugeeism, especially in the initial stages of dislocation, means that people are not in stable situations or environments conducive to thorough needs assessment. Second, the contexts in which refugees are located vary enormously, from large camps, to centres of detainment, or to fringe dwelling in suburban communities in countries of resettlement. This means that the needs of refugee groups are context dependent and are also relative to the stage of refugeeism in which they find themselves. Third, understanding the needs of people who are refugees from an occupational perspective, or indeed any perspective, also means having to acknowledge the impacts of the trauma that many refugees have lived through. The impacts of such trauma may be evident through the presence of post traumatic stress disorder (Sack *et al.*, 1999), anxiety or depression (Howard & Hodes, 2000), and a general reluctance to discuss some issues due to a host of fears and anxieties.

Given these challenges and that there has been relatively little data generated which has sought to uncover the needs of refugees from an occupational perspective, the author instigated some exploratory research. A description of the research, alongside a discussion of some narrative extracts which highlight the occupational issues and needs of two people involved in the study, are presented below.

13.3.1   Uncovering the occupational issues of refugees: a pilot study

In the first quarter of 2002, the author obtained ethics approval from the Charles Sturt University Ethics Committee to conduct a pilot study with people who had been refugees, currently living in the Murray Valley district of New South Wales, Australia. Recruitment took place through members of the local Rural Australians for Refugees Group. Members distributed information sheets on the study and potential participants contacted the author directly.

Once consent processes were explained and consent forms signed, interviews were conducted with the use of a pseudonym chosen by the participant. In one instance, an interpreter was used in the interview, which, as has been previously acknowledged in the literature, added another level of complexity to the interview (Grbich, 1999). All interviews were tape recorded and transcribed and analysis of the narrative data proceeded using open coding technique (De Poy & Gitlin, 1998) and identification of key themes (Grbich, 1999). The key themes identified thus far in the study are presented and discussed below. It should be noted that, as the study has been conducted as an exploratory pilot study, the data presented are tentative and represent the preliminary findings of the study. Trustworthiness has been addressed throughout the study via strategies including peer debriefing, the generation of an audit trail and reflexive processes in the form of a journal (De Poy & Gitlin, 1998). Given the distressing nature of some interview content, peer debriefing has been of particular importance and value to the author.

Mr V.: a case study in occupational deprivation

Mr V. is a middle-aged Albanian man with three children. Previously he lived in a small town in Kosovo, and was a respected teacher with graduate qualifications. He was earning a good salary and his wife was primarily involved in home duties, but also undertook some work in the garment industry. The parents of Mr V. lived close by as did Mrs V.'s mother and there was much family interaction on a daily basis. Mr V. reported that the discrimination against people of Albanian ethnicity in the 1980s began to impact negatively on his work:

> 'Discrimination politics started against normal Albanian people. Increasingly, Albanian students started having schooling in private homes – for Albanian teachers [like me] I end up working in a Serbian programme. The Serbian language is a different language; between Serbian and Albanian, big difference. So, I change jobs. I start working in a furniture factory for five years from '92. At this time there was a big difference in Kosovo – the politics of discrimination – and some people had gone to live in other countries in Europe. By 1997 it was not a good situation in Kosovo.'

From this commentary, it is evident that although we tend to associate disruption and changed life circumstances with dramatic conflict, the political contexts in which people live can subtly influence their lives and patterns of occupational participation for a long period of time beforehand. What Mr V. describes here is the beginning of a long-standing period of occupational disruption and deprivation: he is forced out of his primary role as a teacher which has status and is well remunerated, into work in a furniture factory. As he indicated, this situation was so intolerable for some that they actively relocated.

Mr V. continues his story through the period of time of conflict in Kosovo and his family's experience of fleeing and camp existence in a neighbouring area:

> 'In our camp there were 40 000 people. There was no water, no way of washing, it was very bad, some people were sick, some died. There was no food, no eating. People returned on buses [from the conflict areas], they had been mutilated by knives, guns. The programme was run by the United Nations; people were working day and night for the aid of drink and everything, there was no sleeping. We were all in there together, my mother and father, they're old people. Some people couldn't make it in to eat, the old or sick people, so we helped them, very important to help – all living together, one family. For me, I

was up every morning at five trying to find out which country we would be going to.'

The reflections of Mr V. on the conditions in the UN camp are compelling even though they reflect a reality most of us have never experienced. The combination of trauma, continued fear, cramped quarters, the presence of sick and dying people and the uncertainty of what would happen next, would all appear to contribute to a stressful situation. Indeed, Williams (1990) suggests that the experience of living in camps can be destabilizing, leading to a breakdown in normative social interactions. The fact that many camp residents also suffer from post-traumatic stress disorder also contributes to this situation. From an occupational perspective, however, the reference in Mr V.'s account to the caregiving roles adopted by camp members towards each other is notable. Perhaps taking care of others in this context served not just a pragmatic function, but an occupationally meaningful one as well because, as Frankl's (1997) work reminds us, meanings relate to unique situations and the uniqueness of the individual encountering them. Whilst such interpretations may be possible, they remain at the level of conjecture in the light of too little information on these deeply complex issues. What is evident, is that we

'are limited in our current understanding of the experience of being a refugee in a camp setting. In order to understand both individual and family members' response and coping strategies, a theoretical framework that allows for the analysis of meanings in process is needed.' (Williams, 1990, p. 107)

The time Mr V. and his family spent in a refugee camp in Australia contrasted with their experience in the large UN camp. The Australian camp was one established in the small Victorian town of Porepunka and housed ethnic Albanians who had been victims in the Kosovo conflict. The situation at Porepunka seemed to allow more opportunities for engagement in normative routines and occupations, probably because it was a smaller, more permanent and better resourced facility. Mr V. recounts the types of things that he and his family did that created a sense of community and coherence:

'Porepunka was good, lots of people willing to help. During the day, some people would go and learn English, and the kids would have school. For me, I was teaching the Albanian students in the morning, it was voluntary, not paid or anything, but important for [future] plans ... [also] we could go to the recreation centre, some young people played soccer. Every week we organized music, singing or dancing together, we also cooked Albanian food, pitta and baklava and dolma with yoghurt and garlic plus special salad. We would cook then share our food ... one day some people [from the community] came for lunch for traditional food.'

Whilst the opportunities afforded at Porepunka were much greater and allowed for the Albanian refugee group to establish daily routines and engage in the culturally meaningful occupations of food preparation and music making, it was still a centre where people were detained. Mr V. remembers how they were reminded of their refugee status through media attention and the presence of security

'The name refugee is very hard for some people to understand. Most people in the town were good and wanted to help, but that first day, some people didn't understand and they visited the camp, there was strong security, some journalists with cameras ... this was very upsetting.'

It seems from this description that the experience of being a refugee, being labelled as such and then being made publicly 'other' by being kept in a secure environment, was distressing to Mr V. and his family. The family were eventually sent back to nightmarish Kosovo where they had to reapply to return to Australia. Eventually the family returned to Victoria, where the children entered primary school and Mr V. commenced looking for work.

Whilst Mr V. reports being largely happy to be in Australia, there are still major issues with which he has to contend. First, he and his wife had to leave aged parents behind in Kosovo, who they believe they will never see again. Second, they both need to increase their English language skills in order to engage more fully in occupations within the community at large, or in parenting their children who have become bilingual. Third, Mr V. has so far been unable to find work, which has significant financial implications. He has been unemployed since his return and, like many refugees whilst they are often well qualified, their qualifications are not recognized in their new countries (Iredale, 1994; Lamb, 1995; Stevens, 1996). Whilst language and specific training constitute significant barriers to employment, the attitudes of employers is often problematic (Iredale, 1994) to the extent that it has been described as constituting 'direct, indirect and/ or systematic discrimination' (Stevens, 1996, p. 274). As a corollary to this situation, Mr V. has now travelled to another town in Victoria with a large Albanian community, hoping that he may get part-time work teaching Albanian. It is more likely, however, that he will end up in a menial or semi-skilled position. This is a reality for many male refugees in Australia, evidenced by the fact that during the period 1988–89 for example, whilst 39.1% of male refugees were from managerial, professional or paraprofessional occupations pre-migration, only 5.1% entered these areas in their first occupation in the country of resettlement (Iredale, 1994). Based on these statistics, it is no wonder that 'loss of occupational status might be seen as a significant source of psychological distress in addition to other factors inherent in being a refugee' (Klimidis *et al*, 1991, p. 157).

Routine, communication and connection: Maria's story of resettlement

Maria is a mother of two, who came to Australia following the conflict in Bosnia. The details of Maria's background and the events that led to her arrival are not clear, because at the time of interview Maria was still afraid to disclose any information regarding her past, due to a continuing fear of reprisal and/or persecution. All that I could ascertain was that she had spent some time living in hiding, in dire circumstances, prior to arriving in Australia.

Consequently, the focus of Maria's narrative revolved around her experiences of settling in a town in regional Australia with her two girls, aged six and eight. Their story is a compelling one that underscores some of the very real challenges refugee families face in their attempts to reconstruct their lives in a new country. As is evident from the following account, the first year of resettlement is particularly demanding, not least because re-engaging in familiar occupations and routines is difficult in a very different environment:

'The first year is the most difficult time, because you have left behind your family, your friends, your home and then you come here and it's absolutely, you come into the unknown. You can't speak the language, you don't know the people, you don't know the place, that's very difficult. Despite the fact that the volunteer people that were around us were very good and wanted to help, it was difficult. I remember the first shopping we went to the supermarket and of course don't know any of the products and what they are, and, for example, I said I wanted flour and tea, and the lady who was helping me with the shopping she was trying to tell me to get self raising flour and I'd never used self raising flour in our country. I wanted ordinary flour and could not understand why she wanted me to use something that they used here and I hadn't used. So, after that first shopping they did for me, I felt like throwing everything in the rubbish because there was nothing I could use, nothing was familiar to me.'

This is a poignant account of how an everyday occupation such as shopping for groceries becomes a frustrating exercise in an unfamiliar domain. It is possible that shopping for groceries is actually a precursor to being able to re-engage in a valued and familiar occupation of Maria's, that of cooking, but that the lack of familiar ingredients represented a barrier. Such frustrations seem to breed a desire for the familiar, a phenomenon also apparently echoed by Maria's two girls who she describes as begging her to 'Cook Bosnian food, please. Cook Bosnian meat!' Additionally, this description points to the importance of the objects with which we interact in order to engage in occupations of meaning (Hocking, 1997) and how changes in occupational form impact on perceived satisfaction and meaning (Nelson, 1988). In Maria's case, it is also possible that the very difference of the items is symbolic of the culturally different milieu in which she now finds herself.

In terms of daily routine, Maria further expands on some of the difficulties she encountered in trying to re-establish familiar occupations for herself and her daughters and posits some suggestions as to how this could be ameliorated for other refugees in the early phase of resettlement:

'What I felt was that although they gave me some volunteer people to look after me and help me out, it wasn't necessary to have this many people around and most of the ladies were older than me and I found their way of thinking different to mine. They had different routines than what I had and I felt that they didn't really match, they were used to a different way of life. It would have been better if there was one family looking after another family, as it was in my case, there were older ladies; one came to my place and she would sit down for three or four hours but we couldn't communicate, we couldn't talk. Then someone else would come with something else ... The trouble was we had to walk a long distance from the flat to the school and because I was also studying [English] I'd sit until the older girl came home from school, but then maybe the little one would go to sleep – there was no routine.'

That daily and weekly routines are pivotal to occupational engagement, is a proposition that has been held for some time now in occupational therapy. Most recently, Kielhofner (2002, p. 68) suggests that routines 'create the overall pattern by which we go about our various occupations.'

For Maria, it seems that her attempts to reconstruct her life in Australia necessarily began with the creation of the superstructure of everyday living: routine. In her early efforts, however, she struggled to do this in the presence of a well-meaning army of volunteers whose comings and goings actually mitigated against the development of a daily routine. Her suggestion then, of a family 'buddied' system appears to have merit. Living close to another family would facilitate the naturalistic development of a routine through a staged process, namely one in which initially daily routines and occupations of the host family and new family are meshed to an extent. This would then progress through the development of parallel, but supported, routine structures, moving to the con-solidation of a daily routine that is somewhere between interdependent and independent depending on the relationship between the families.

Clearly, these are the sorts of insights that emerge from first hand experience and should inform refugee resettlement policy. Maria also acknowledges that the situation of each refugee is different and that perhaps solutions should be based on an acknowledgement of that difference:

'We are all different. For every case it's a different situation. Everybody has a different experience because some people might come and stay with their families or friends and then some people might come over and be accepted by a group of volunteers. Some people come with money, some with no money and then some might have a person that speaks a bit of English. Most of them have that same process of trying to learn English, but if they've learned in their country then they have some knowledge.'

One of the themes highlighted in the extract above is that the ability to com-municate in the language of the host country is a common challenge to all refu-gees, whatever their backgrounds. For many refugees the demands of resettlement alongside the acquisition of a new language is a daunting prospect and one that has been identified as a real stressor (Driver & Beltran, 1998). Lan-guage competence is in many ways central to social integration and occupational participation and is especially crucial in obtaining employment (Klimidis *et al.*, 1991; Ethnic Youth Issues Network, 1999). Maria concurs:

'The worst thing is the language . . . I find it hard as I end up sitting at home, and though we'd like to go somewhere we can't because I can't read the map and it's just very difficult. It's probably impossible, but the first thing I would like to do is master the language and then I would like to have a job.'

As well as finding English competency a challenge in seeking employment, Maria also acknowledges how a lack of extended family in her new country makes getting a job more difficult. This is very possibly true for many refugees and points to the need for support mechanisms within communities:

'It would be nice to have somebody like a family member that I could leave the children with when, maybe I could find a part-time job, some sort of work, though now they're too young to be left as well . . . it's totally different in Bosnia . . . what would be good would be to have the conditions we live in here with the child rearing practices we have in Bosnia.'

The focus of Maria's reflections in the extract above points to the complex set of interrelated factors that mitigate against occupational participation. Refugees arriving in new countries not only have to deal with the structural dimensions of their host environments, such as dwelling arrangements and co-location of extended family members, but also with deeply embedded cultural practices, such as the example given here of child rearing. The discussion of the extended family and their role in enabling patterns of occupational engagement for each other is relatively poorly understood due to a lack of focused research into occupation as a culturally relative concept (Whiteford & Wilcock, 2000). However, notwithstanding this fact, Maria's narrative also suggests that contact with others, especially extended family, is also important to a sense of connectedness, of 'being' and its relationship to doing (Wilcock, 1999).

Here Maria expands on the differences in feeling connected to others between Bosnia and Australia:

'It's different there. You know there could be ten villages and you know people from the tenth village and when somebody comes for a visit everybody knows them and it's like a big family ... the neighbourhoods were a lot safer back home, you didn't have to walk everywhere with your kids, the people in the neighbourhood know each other and help each other, but here you don't ... everybody needs friends and family around and it's particularly hard here in holiday time and the kids are home and it's difficult because there's no family to go to, no family circle, and I remember when we first came here once, the kids said to me, "why did we come here when there is none of our family here?"'

In closing, Maria reflects on what she sees as the trade off between having the sense of connectedness to and support of others, and the opportunities afforded by a new country:

'Back home we wouldn't have such a good life as we have here. Maybe we have the family, but we wouldn't have this sort of life so I had to choose and I had to give something up and I had to give up the family and have a better life, and so the children can have a better life.'

In summary, while Maria's story of refugeeism and resettlement is unique, a number of themes apparent in her narrative may well reflect the experiences of others. The challenge of recreating a life in a new country following the often traumatic flight from the country of origin is significant and potentially over-whelming. From Maria's account, the process of attempting to re-engage in everyday occupations is difficult in the new country because of a number of factors. These include:

- Language and the isolation that can accompany a lack of language competence.
- The diminished opportunities for occupational participation in both paid employment and leisure occupations, due to language difficulties and financial status.
- The difficulties associated with developing and maintaining a routine in an unfamiliar environment.
- The lack of both pragmatic and emotional support afforded by the presence of family.
- The absence of a sense of 'connectedness' to others in the community due to the socio-cultural and environmental differences between the two countries.

The identification of these factors mentioned in the narrative accounts of people such as Maria, should help inform policy and programme initiatives in the area of refugee resettlement. Whilst Mr V.'s experiences may also echo these themes, his particular story highlights the complex process of occupational disruption that can begin for refugees as a result of conflict, alienation or persecution in their home country, long before they are forced to leave. The experiences of Mr V. and his family in camps both in Macedonia and Australia provide useful information regarding the naturalistic, occupational responses of refugees living within them. Clearly, at both ends of the continuum of the process of refugeeism, the needs and issues of people living through these experiences go beyond merely a requirement for safety, food and shelter. They indicate a need to respond to the trauma and uncertainty through the active engagement in meaningful occupation both during containment, and later in resettlement. How these needs can be addressed by occupational therapists is the focus of the next section of this chapter.

13.4   Occupationally focused action and interventions

Based on a review of related literature and the needs of people who have lived through the experience of being a refugee, there are a number of potential areas for occupationally focused action. These have been identified as being at two distinct points in the process of refugeeism: in refugee camps and in host country resettlement programmes.

13.4.1   Refugee camps

'Camps can serve their purpose well where they are prevented from becoming militarized, where the rule of law is maintained, where adequate health care, education and other essential services are provided and where refugees have an opportunity to sustain themselves. It is to these ends that humanitarian efforts should be focused.' (UNHCR, 2000, p. 109)

Although there exists some debate as to whether self settlement or camp settlement in a host country is more desirable, the fact is that the number of refugee camps established internationally since the 1980s has increased, with host countries being motivated to establish camps because of their visibility and ability to attract international aid assistance (UNHCR, 2000). Occupationally focused action, within general relief programmes, could take the form of the following:

Environmental adaptation
Securing or developing sites within the camp in which subgroups of refugees can naturalistically engage in occupations and co-occupations together. For example, space for children to play and women to gather whilst performing occupations.

Routine development
Assisting in the development of a daily/weekly routine within the camp in order to minimize disorientation and enhance occupational adaptation. This would include the scheduling of events at set and appropriate times.

Enhancing opportunities for engagement in self-care and caregiving
Creating an environment in which the refugee residents are able to engage in the everyday occupations of self-care, food preparation, child rearing etc. in culturally appropriate ways. Given the number of people living in camps without family members, facilitating naturalistic patterns of caregiving to and interaction with, children, people with injuries and disabilities, and the aged, is potentially beneficial to both caregiver and recipient.

Creating opportunities for economic self-sufficiency
Facilitating projects through which long-term camp residents can engage in activities which, in interaction with the local community, have the potential to be income generating. An example of such activity was the Khao-I-Dang camp in Thailand in which Cambodian refugees ran food stalls and a bicycle transport service (UNHCR, 2000).

13.4.2   Resettlement programmes

'Refugees are unlike other migrants in that they are forced to move, they have no option They arrive unprepared for resettlement ... [Australia] needs to do more than select people and then leave them to their own devices. Carefully planned and ongoing programmes are needed to help refugees integrate successfully.' (Iredale, 1994, p. 241).

As suggested in this cogent quote from Iredale, resettlement programmes need to be planned, coordinated and resourced on an ongoing basis. A focus on maximizing the occupational participation of refugees could include, depending on the existing refugee resettlement policies of the new host country, the following:

- Facilitating identification of and interaction with, refugee families and groups from similar backgrounds, in the form of a formalized buddy system.
- Facilitating community and social participation through use of pre-existing structures and facilities.
- Designing and developing skills-based educational programmes for refugee adults and youth.
- Facilitating the creation of community focused employment solutions.

13.5   Future roles and directions

Adopting an occupational perspective in addressing the needs of refugees, whatever stage of the process they are at, need not necessarily be limited to direct intervention. Indeed, longer-term impacts on the quality of life of refugees require a range of roles at many levels. These include extending the knowledge base through researching the occupational needs and occupational adjustment strategies of refugees; advocating for the rights of asylum seekers and refugees; educating others as to the needs and rights of asylum seekers and refugees; and shaping refugee policy through lobbying submission writing. A brief discussion of each of these roles precedes the conclusion to this chapter.

Researcher

Despite the fact that there has been a dramatic increase in the number of asylum seekers and refugees globally, there has been relatively little focused research in the area of the occupational needs and strategies of refugees either in camps, in self or supported settlement. This is very possibly due to a number of factors, not least of which is, in the camp situation, the pragmatic constraints of conducting research in often hostile environments and, in the host country, of accessing refugee communities. However, notwithstanding such constraints, we desperately need to understand more about the impacts of and responses to refugeeism, in order to better address the needs of people at varying stages of the experience. Naturalistic, non-invasive research approaches and methods are clearly indicated in this field, due to the sensitive nature of the issues and concerns of the possible participants as well as their potential vulnerability. Action methods which involve stakeholder groups such as refugee representative organizations and aid agencies would be the approach of choice in order to most quickly inform policy and programme planning.

Advocate

Refugees are often marginalized in the countries in which they seek refuge because of their lack of language skills, their relatively low levels of occupational participation in the community at large and their corresponding lack of representation in key forums. For asylum seekers, the situation in many countries is even worse, especially where they are forcibly detained and have no freedom of communication or movement. As professionals, occupational therapists are well positioned to act as important advocates on refugee and asylum seekers' rights. In fact, it could be argued that we are professionally mandated to play such a role, given the profession's very early roots in the pursuit of social justice (Wilcock, 2001). Advocacy in this area has been made more possible through the emergence of a number of groups and networks in most developed countries which play a key role in highlighting the needs of refugees. In Australia, a particularly successful example has been the formation of the Rural Australians for Refugees network which highlights the fact that economically, as well as socially and culturally, rural Australia can benefit from the presence of skilled refugees into population-depleted areas.

Educator

Generally speaking, there is still a relatively poor understanding of the issues surrounding asylum seekers and refugees in many countries. This is due in part to the scare tactics often adopted by local media with respect to the coverage of refugee issues and reinforced by the lack of basic information regarding, for example, what constitutes a refugee as opposed to an asylum seeker. As professionals with an ability to access and influence media, occupational therapists have opportunities to help educate the public at large as to the needs, occupational and otherwise, of refugees and highlight their situation. Publishing at a range of levels, from newsletter through to refereed journal, is also a means of raising awareness of refugee concerns and initiating possible actions by communities and professional groups on their behalf.

Lobbyist

Ultimately, the decision making process regarding asylum seekers and refugees whether in camps, detention centres or in resettlement programmes is a political one. Occupational therapists, as individuals and as a professional group, can lobby key figures in the policy arena on important issues in the refugee debate, especially highlighting the need to recognize the occupational needs of refugees at all stages of the process. Strategic lobbying activities coupled with focused submission writing in key areas can be instrumental to policy changes, legislative action and the resource decisions of governments. Clearly, this is an important arena for us to be active in, to highlight the needs and rights of refugees.

13.6   Conclusion

This chapter has discussed refugeeism around the globe in the new millennium. In attempting to highlight the occupational issues and needs of refugees, some narrative data from a pilot study of refugees undertaken in Australia has been presented and discussed from an occupational perspective. This data, along with the literature in the area, has informed the identification of key areas of involvement for occupationally focused action and future roles for occupational therapists.

It is hoped that this chapter has also highlighted three important ideas. First, the world's number of asylum seekers and refugees is increasing and this requires global acknowledgement, planning and subsequent action. Second, the issues of refugees are largely occupational in nature and can be addressed through focused action and intervention, and through the adoption of a number of roles and strategies. Third, and most importantly, occupational therapists are ideally placed to play a lead role in addressing refugees' needs because of their unique occupational perspective. In doing so, the profession would not only be tackling one of the biggest challenges of the present and future, but it would also be honouring its historic commitment to social justice, a tradition which must remain at the forefront of our endeavours whichever era we collectively find ourselves in.

References

De Poy, E. & Gitlin, L. (1998). *Introduction to Research: Understanding and Applying Multiple Strategies*. St Louis: Mosby.

Driver, C. & Beltran, R. (1998). Impact of refugee trauma on children's occupational role as school student. *Australian Occupational Therapy Journal, 45*, 23–38.

Ethnic Youth Issues Network (1999). Putting educational pathways for refugee and migrant young people back on the agenda. *Migration Action, 21* (3), 35–40.

Frankl, V. (1997). *Man's Search for Ultimate Meaning*. Reading: Perseus.

Garner, R. (2001). Asylum seekers are educated and skilled. *The Independent*, 28 June: Retrieved 16 July, 2002, from
http://www.unhcr.ch/cgi-bin/texis/vtx/print?tbl=NEWS&id=3b3c48b44

Goodwin-Gill, G. (1996). *The Refugee in International Law*. Oxford: Oxford University Press.

Grbich, C. (1999). *Qualitative Research in Health*. St. Leonards, NSW: Allen & Unwin.

Hocking, C. (1997). Person object interaction model: understanding the use of everyday objects. *Journal of Occupational Science, 4* (1), 27–33.

Howard, M. & Hodes, M. (2000). Psychopathology, adversity and service utilization of young refugees. *Journal of the American Academy of Child & Adolescent Psychiatry, 39* (3), 368–377.

Iredale, R. (1994). Skills recognition and refugees: migrants without options. *Australian Journal of Social Issues, 29* (3), 241–264.

Jupp, J. (2002). The pacific solution. *Dialogue, 21* (1), 10–15.

Kielhofner, G. (2002). Habituation: patterns of daily occupation. In: G. Kielhofner (Ed.), *A Model of Human Occupation: Theory and Application* (pp. 63–80). Baltimore: Lippincott Williams & Wilkins.

Klimidis, S., Lien, O. & Minas, I.H. (1991). Vietnamese presenting to a bilingual psychiatric service: demographic and diagnostic characteristics. In: I.H. Minas (Ed.), *Cultural Diversity and Mental Health. Proceedings of the 14th Annual Symposium of the Section of Social and Cultural Psychiatry.* Sydney: Royal Australian and New Zealand College of Psychiatrists.

Lamb, C. (1995). Refugee women in Australia: the relationship between employment status and mental health. Proceedings of the 3rd National Women's Health Conference. Canberra.

Loff, B. (2002). Detention of asylum seekers in Australia. *The Lancet, 359*, 792–793.

McMaster, D. (2002). Refugees: Where to now? *Dialogue, 21* (1), 3–8.

Nelson, D. (1988). Occupation: form and performance. *American Journal of Occupational Therapy, 42* (10), 633–641.

Pittaway, E. & Bartolomei, L. (2002). Refugees, race and gender: the multiple discrimination against refugee women. *Dialogue, 21* (1), 16–27.

Sack, W., Him, C. & Dickason, D. (1999). Twelve-year follow-up of Khmer youths who suffered massive war trauma as children. *Journal of the American Academy of Child & Adolescent Psychiatry, 38* (9), 1173–1179.

Schnyder, F. (1962). Statement by Mr Felix Schnyder, United Nations High Commissioner for Refugees, to the Third (Social, Humanitarian and Cultural) Committee of the General Assembly on 19 November 1962. Retrieved 16 July, 2002, from www.unhcr.ch/cgi-bin/texts/

Sidoti, C. (2002). Refugee policy: is there a way out of this mess? *Dialogue, 21* (1), 28–41.

Silove, D. & Steel, Z. (1998). *The Mental Health & Well-Being of On-shore Asylum Seekers in Australia.* Sydney, NSW: Psychiatry and Research Training Unit.

Smith, M. (2001). Asylum seekers in Australia. *Medical Journal of Australia, 175*, 587–589.

Stevens, C. (1996). The labour market experience of Cambodians: policy implications for settlement services. *Australian Journal of Social Issues, 31* (3), 271–299.

Sultan, A. & O'Sullivan, K. (2001). Psychological disturbances in asylum seekers held in long-term detention: a participant-observer account. *Medical Journal of Australia, 175*, 593–596.

United Nations High Commission for Refugees (2000). *The State of the World's Refugees.* Oxford: Oxford University Press.

United Nations High Commission for Refugees (2002a). Basic facts. Retrieved 16 July 2002 from http://www.unhcr.ch/cgi-bin/texis/vtx/basics

United Nations High Commission for Refugees (2002b). Global consultations on international protection: refugee women. Retrieved 16 July 2002 from www.unhcr.ch/cgi-bin/texts/vtx/home

Whiteford, G. & Wilcock, A. (2000). Cultural relativism: occupation and independence reconsidered. *Canadian Journal of Occupational Therapy, 67* (5), 324–336.

Wilcock, A. A. (1999). Reflections on doing, being and becoming. *Australian Occupational Therapy Journal, 46* (1), 1–11.

Wilcock, A. (2001). *Occupation for Health. Volume 1: A Journey from Self Health to Prescription.* London: College of Occupational Therapists.

Williams, H.A. (1990). Families in refugee camps. *Human Organisation, 49* (2), 100–109.

Chapter 14
Occupational Science, Occupational Therapy and Evidence-based Practice: What the Well Elderly Study has Taught Us

Florence A. Clark, Jeanne Jackson and Mike Carlson

14.1 Introduction

It is over a decade since we received funding to undertake the University of Southern California (USC) Well Elderly Study in 1993 (Clark *et al.*, 1997; Jackson *et al.*, 1998; Clark *et al.*, 2001; Hay *et al.*, 2002), and so it seems appropriate to take stock of what we have learned from the experience of conducting the largest randomized clinical trial to date, in the history of occupational therapy. Many of the lessons we have gleaned could have been anticipated, but others were totally unexpected.

In this chapter, first we summarize the findings of the USC Well Elderly Study in the light of current enthusiasm for evidence-based practice. Next, we discuss what we feel were the particular facets of the lifestyle intervention that created the positive results. We then map out practice applications as well as new directions that our work has taken since the completion of the Well Elderly Study. In the last section, we discuss what we have identified as some of the best strategies for preparing students and clinicians to apply lifestyle redesign interventions.

14.2 Overview: the USC Well Elderly Study

14.2.1 An evidence-based practice approach

Evidence-based practice is defined as 'integrating individual clinical expertise' with the 'conscientious, explicit and judicious use of current best evidence in making decisions about the care of individual patients' (Sackett *et al.*, 1996, p. 71). Although the ideal of evidence-based practice is widely recognized by occupational therapists, leading researchers in the field point out that only a few intervention approaches have been researched thoroughly enough to enable confident appraisal of their effectiveness (Law & Baum, 1998; Tickle-Degnen, 1999; Holm, 2000; Christiansen & Lou, 2001). According to Sackett *et al.* (1996), randomized clinical trials are one of the strongest forms of evidence available for establishing the effectiveness of an intervention.

At USC, our favoured approach to evidence-based practice has been to conduct occupational science-based clinical trials (Table 14.1 depicts this strategy). Our intent, as exemplified in the Well Elderly Study, is to employ preliminary basic research to provide groundwork leading to the development of a carefully conceived therapeutic model to be tested within the trial. Follow-through in the form of assessing the intervention's long-term effects and cost implications is also incorporated, with an eye toward dissemination of study findings and training of therapists to promote widespread application of the intervention after the trial is completed.

Table 14.1 Strategy for doing evidenced-based practice in occupational science

Step 1	Conduct literature review and perform basic research (usually in the form of pilot studies) in occupational science to gain a comprehensive understanding of the considerations that must be taken into account to design an optimal intervention.
Step 2	Modify existing occupational therapy best practice models in accord with the results of step one.
Step 3	Conduct a carefully designed randomized clinical trial through collaboration with clinicians to determine the efficacy of the intervention.
Step 4	Conduct follow-up and cost-effectiveness studies on the intervention.
Step 5	Disseminate findings and train clinicians in the intervention approach.

It is important to note that we view the above strategy as only one among many viable methods for promoting evidence-based practice. Because our approach includes preliminary basic research to better understand the link between occupation and health in the targeted treatment population, outcomes pertaining to the intervention may unfold at a somewhat slower pace than is usual in clinical trials. However, by gathering previously unavailable information, novel findings emerge that have the potential to deepen our understanding of occupation's link to health in the target population, thereby spawning important therapeutic innovations. While it is legitimate to examine an existing treatment protocol in the absence of basic scientific spadework, our alternate approach is complementary in that it opens the door for the derivation and assessment of novel techniques.

The Well Elderly Study was our first attempt to enact this strategy. In 1993, when our research team received US National Institutes of Health (NIH) funding to conduct the Well Elderly Study, we were a bit daunted. What if this rigorous test of the effectiveness of occupational therapy showed no treatment effect? The fact that the design of the study enabled comparison of a professionally led occupational therapy programme not only to a no-treatment control condition, but also to a non-professionally led activity programme, meant that we would be subjecting occupational therapy to an exceedingly stringent test of its efficacy. Initially hesitant to proceed, ultimately our research group decided to embark on the study, convinced that the likelihood of showing a positive effect was high, given the care with which we had hammered out the research design and our strong intuitive sense that occupational therapy was effective. Additionally, we were committed to the principle that the science would reveal outcomes worth pursuing no matter what results surfaced. Further, we reasoned that if the results were positive occupational therapists worldwide would be injected with confidence.

It took three years to complete the trial, which required that two-thirds of the 361 participants undergo nine months of intervention. The ethnically diverse elderly participants were randomly assigned to one of three groups: (1) a nine-month programme of group-based occupational therapy focusing on lifestyle redesign; (2) a control condition involving participation in non-professionally led group-based activities; or (3) no treatment whatsoever. The study results were powerful and consistent. In comparison to the control conditions, occupational therapy produced solid benefits in numerous outcome domains including vitality, physical functioning, social functioning and mental health (Clark *et al.*, 1997). Moreover, in contrast to the short-lived effects of most interventions for ageing populations, the benefits of occupational therapy persisted over a six-month follow-up interval, in the absence of further treatment (Clark *et al.*, 2001).

Additionally, in our most recent analysis (Hay *et al.*, 2002), we provided evidence that the experimental intervention (lifestyle redesign) achieved its results in a financially effective way. Based on interview data collected on the research participants' health-related expenditures, a trend was observed for substantially reduced health care costs for the elders who underwent the occupational therapy intervention (relative to elders in the two control groups). In fact, the average savings over time in health care costs exceeded the cost of therapy itself, suggesting that preventive occupational therapy has the ability to simultaneously improve elders' health and save money to health care providers.

Further, to test the cost-effectiveness of the intervention, a technical index of overall quality of life gain (quality adjusted life year or QALY) was computed to determine whether the benefits were achieved in a sufficiently inexpensive manner. Generally speaking, interventions that cost US$50 000 or less per QALY gain are considered cost-effective. Using this criterion, the lifestyle redesign occupational therapy intervention was found to be highly successful, requiring less than US$11 000 per QALY gain when compared to control conditions. As economist Joel Hay has pointed out, 'We held the treatment up against the industry standard for measuring cost-effectiveness, comparing it to therapies such as heart bypass surgery and breast cancer chemotherapy. We demonstrated that occupational therapy is an enormous value for the money' (Preidt, 2002). The net result of our latest research findings is that not only can occupational therapy enhance the health and quality of life of the growing population of older adults, but that it can also play a crucial role in reducing the huge burden in elder health care costs that looms on the horizon.

14.2.2   Why was lifestyle redesign so effective?

As we have not yet conducted a follow-up study on the precise mechanisms that account for the positive results of the Well Elderly lifestyle redesign intervention, at this point we can only present our thoughts on this by highlighting six key aspects of the programme. The reader is reminded, however, that we offer only provisional hypotheses.

Grounding in occupational science

The first is that the design of the programme was derived from occupational science, although it also capitalized on techniques and approaches that comprise traditional occupational therapy. A key point here is that in conducting this study we followed the steps depicted in Table 14.1. First, we conducted basic research in occupational science that led to the way in which the intervention protocol was manualized. Our challenge was to design a protocol for the local target group our study was to address, one that had the greatest chance of being maximally effective. To settle upon an intervention design, not only did we review the relevant literature but, in addition, we conducted preliminary qualitative basic research to gain a fuller understanding of the kinds of adaptive strategies used by elders similar to those whom we planned to recruit for the trial. Results of this initial study (Clark *et al.*, 1996a) were vital for identification of the domains that eventually comprised the lifestyle redesign intervention and for enhancing our knowledge of potential adaptive strategies elders could use to lead happier and healthier lives.

When a researcher conducts a clinical trial he or she can evaluate practice as it is currently done, assess the effectiveness of entirely new interventions based on current findings in basic research, or evaluate interventions that are a hybrid of both (i.e. that include elements of traditional practice, but with modification in light of current basic and other research). The lifestyle redesign intervention was hybrid in that it emphasized elements of traditional occupational therapy practice such as 'safety', but also included modules such as 'cultural issues and occupation' derived from our basic research (see Clark *et al.*, 1996a). We believe that it is often necessary to do evidence-based research on current practice, and in such cases it is not necessary to do the preliminary basic research. However, there is a danger in restricting the majority of occupational therapy outcome studies to these kinds of studies.

Imagine, for example, that status quo practice (i.e. practice as it is typically done) is shown to be ineffective. New or modified approaches would then be needed to revitalize the profession. If they are informed by cutting-edge basic research on occupation, such interventions stand the maximum chance of being effective. In point of fact, our research group decided to concentrate on studying the effectiveness of hybrid interventions, leaving it to other groups to provide evidence of the effectiveness of more traditional therapeutic approaches.

Cultural sensitivity

The second reason we believe the Well Elderly intervention was so effective is because it was culturally sensitized for the diverse population that resided at Angelus Plaza and Pilgrim Tower, the two low-income senior housing projects in Los Angeles from which we recruited participants. Those who have read the study will know that 47% of the participants in the study were Asian American and of these 31% spoke only Mandarin Chinese. As a consequence, we used systematic qualitative procedures to add a second language to the study protocol and provide culturally sensitive health care (Jackson *et al.*, 2000). Because we surmised that both body language as well as the second language itself could potentially hinder communication and threaten therapeutic relationships, we enacted numerous modifications to adapt the lifestyle redesign programme for the Mandarin population.

A bilingual, bicultural research team had to be recruited, including testers, coordinators, instrument translators, a programme adaptation team, occupational therapists and social (activity) programme leaders. But perhaps most importantly, we undertook a rigorous process through which the treatment protocol was rendered culturally sensitive. (See Jackson *et al.*, 2000, for a detailed description of the procedures.) The programme adaptation team consisted of individuals we refer to as 'culture brokers'. They were individuals who had in-depth experiences in Mandarin Chinese values, language and lifestyle and had the capacity to critique the original lifestyle redesign programme in the light of their sophisticated knowledge of the Mandarin Chinese culture. They also possessed excellent English language skills as well as a nuanced understanding of American culture.

To facilitate adaptation of the treatment for Chinese elders, we first interviewed the culture brokers to obtain information about the relevance of the treatment programme in relation to the needs of the prospective Chinese participants, and then provisionally modified the programme to incorporate this information. We then re-interviewed the culture brokers to verify the appropriateness of the protocol revisions, with discussion continuing until all of the three culture brokers agreed that the protocol was acceptable. The adapted protocol was then administered in the Well Elderly Study, with the therapists soliciting feedback to make further adjustments, leading to a more refined version.

The above process resulted in changes in terms and strategies for handling group dynamics and the ways in which information was presented. For example, instead of using the Mandarin translation of the term 'health', we substituted the phrase 'good for you'. We also developed strategies for showing respect appropriately and impacting knowledge through storytelling rather than a lecture format.

Holistic emphasis on occupation

The third reason we believe that the intervention was so successful is that it emphasized overall lifestyle design rather than specific tasks or activities. We found that for many of the participants the idea of occupation and lifestyle redesign was 'hypo-cognized', meaning, that these concerns in their lives tended to be taken for granted with no deliberation or conscious reflection upon their impact on health, quality of life or ability to promote a meaningful existence. Initially, most elders were virtually unaware of the relationship of occupation to health and tended not to think much about what they were doing each day and how their choices were affecting their physical and mental health, much less their longevity or quality of life. In this regard, an important component of the intervention consisted of allowing the participants to internalize the importance of occupation in their lives.

Just as early in the twentieth century, when occupational therapists focused on enabling people who had been institutionalized to engage in a customary round of daily activities that would be fulfilling and promote health, the therapists who conducted the lifestyle redesign intervention enabled the elders to enact more healthy and satisfying daily routines. We believe this change was possible because through the intervention the elders came to appreciate the importance of doing productive, physical and social activities as a means of staying healthy. They began to strategize overtly so that they could lead richer and more challenging lives. Within sessions, they were able to pinpoint workable solutions for overcoming obstacles and fears, capitalizing on the energy they had, and experiencing greater balance, flexibility and meaning as they engaged in their worlds of occupations. Rather than being mired in a feeling of stagnation, they were able to regain the sense that their lives were moving forward.

Programme structure

The fourth potential reason for the consistent therapeutic effect had to do with the structure of the lifestyle redesign programme (Jackson *et al.*, 1998; Mandel *et al.*, 1999). First, the programme content was derived from a carefully designed needs assessment and was tailored to the needs of the local population we would be studying (Clark *et al.*, 1996a). Moreover, as we have noted, this content was also modified to be culturally sensitive (Jackson *et al.*, 2000). But beyond its content, we believe the programme was successful because of the four modes of delivery that ideally should constitute all lifestyle redesign interventions: didactic presentation, peer exchange, direct experience and personal exploration.

The didactic component involved the therapist conveying content to do with healthy ageing and occupation for each module, through a lecture format. As this content was imparted in groups of 8–10 participants, each participant had the opportunity to contribute to the presentation by injecting his or her insights about the subject matter. Often these peer exchanges would involve one group member offering encouragement to another. The direct experience component was another key ingredient. Not only did the lifestyle redesign programme involve lecture and peer exchange but it was a 'doing' therapy and not simply a 'talking' therapy. Within the programme, participants would go on group excursions accompanied by the therapist to 'try out' the new strategies for living that they had been learning about. This opportunity for active application seemed crucial for the lifestyle redesign intervention to be effective. The fourth method of delivery, personal exploration, provided an opportunity for the elders to reflect upon, make sense of and identify new insights that emerged as a consequence of experiencing the excursions.

We believe that lifestyle redesign was efficacious because it combined group and individualized therapy. During the weekly group the participants experienced content exposure, peer support and interpersonal exchange. In individualized sessions, they were afforded the opportunity to customize the skills they were mastering in relation to their unique life situations. In the end participants were helped to devise a customized plan of daily activity that they could sustain, based on information they accessed and experiences they had in their groups. It is our belief that individualization was crucial (Clark *et al.*, 1997).

Emphasis on habit formation

The fact that the intervention stressed habit formation was a fifth ingredient that made it so effective. As many of you will recall, occupational therapy pioneer Eleanor Clarke Slagle emphasized habit training in the founding days of the profession (Slagle, 1921). Similarly, a key element of the lifestyle redesign treatment was that the nine-month intervention was not only aimed at skill development such as overt strategizing about what to do each day, but also targeted habit formation and inculcation. Elders were taught about and gained experience in healthy lifestyle practices. They also underwent a process of occupational self-analysis through which they performed a personal inventory of their goals, strengths, interests, patterns of activity and weaknesses. They then brought the two together into a customized daily routine that eventually became a habit. It is our feeling that because these routines were realistic, individualized and became habits, they were sustained at the time of follow-up and accounted for the positive effects six months after the intervention ended.

Coaching component

Finally, we speculate that the intervention succeeded because of the way in which therapists served as coaches. In training the therapists who delivered the experimental intervention, we stressed a particular kind of therapeutic use of self. Drawing from Clark (1993) and her colleagues' work (Clark *et al.*, 1996b) on occupational storymaking and storytelling, the therapists were encouraged to see themselves as collaborators with and coaches for the elders in their groups. Techniques and approaches such as active listening, coaching, marking progress and building empathy (Peloquin, 1995) were emphasized. The reader is referred to Mandel *et al.* (1999), Clark (1993) and Clark *et al.* (1996b), for a detailed discussion of these techniques.

14.3   Recent developments in lifestyle redesign

Because the lifestyle redesign approach incorporates basic science principles of personally relevant occupation in relation to health, it potentially extends to numerous populations who either face significant challenges or seek to improve their health. Below, we describe several of the ways that we have attempted to extend the Well Elderly results.

14.3.1   Senior housing communities

As described in the manual entitled *Lifestyle Redesign: Implementing the Well Elderly Programme* (Mandel *et al.*, 1999), following the Well Elderly Study we implemented lifestyle redesign programmes at two assisted-living senior housing communities, both comprised largely of high-income elders. The needs assessments we undertook for these projects are described in the manual in some detail and illustrate the steps that were taken to modify the intervention to be more suitable for the residents of these settings. Of particular interest is the way in which the intervention had to be tailored for an assisted-living programme at one of these settings. We found, for example, that residents in this setting tended not to address one another by name, had poor short-term memories, and often focused on activities only when they were doing them, rather than strategically combining activities, as had been the case in independent living settings. This assisted-living version of the programme, therefore, contained modules that explicitly emphasized the names and unique identities of the participants and activities, and modules that fostered quality of life in the present. At the second setting, the target group was high-income elders who, in most cases, had been in professions or in corporate leadership positions before retirement and had experienced the benefit of higher education. The lifestyle redesign programme we implemented at this setting, therefore, tapped the professional, intellectual and aesthetic tastes of these elders. As much as possible it afforded them the opportunity to be placed in a position of control and, in fact, took on the ambience of an exclusive club. This aspect once again underscores the importance of attending to local variations in the treatment populations.

14.3.2   Prevention of pressure sores in the spinal cord injured population

In 1999, two years after the primary results of the Well Elderly Study had been published, our research group began exploring the applicability of the lifestyle redesign approach with a traditional rehabilitation population. We therefore partnered with clinicians at Rancho Los Amigos National Rehabilitation Centre to conceptualize a research project of this kind. After much discussion, our team of occupational therapy practitioners, physicians, and researchers concluded that the population of people with spinal cord injury who have recurrent, serious

pressure sores would constitute one group for whom a lifestyle redesign programme is much needed and may be extremely cost-effective. Within the United
States, pressure ulcers result in huge medical expenses with the cost of surgery
exceeding US$60 000 per ulcer (Wharton *et al.*, 1987). Further, the national cost of
healing them is estimated at US$1.2 billion annually (Byrne & Salzberg, 1996).
Moreover, tied to this are ethical issues related to who is a good candidate for
surgery (Maynard, 1996).

After a thorough review of the extant literature on the factors that lead to
pressure sore development and the effectiveness of current interventions, we
concluded that before undertaking a randomized clinical trial we needed to
pursue basic occupational science research to better understand the role of daily
occupation in the genesis of pressure ulcers. In fact, this decision meant that we
would, once again, anticipate taking similar steps to those we had taken to prepare for the USC Well Elderly Study, as depicted in Table 14.1. Our review of the
literature revealed that while numerous factors, such as skin type, substance
abuse, activity levels, employment and compliance with pressure release techniques, had been implicated as contributing influences, many of the research
findings were inconsistent or otherwise inconclusive. Further, none of the existing
interventions on which effectiveness studies had been done seemed both powerful and realistically feasible enough to decrease the rates of pressure sore
recurrence.

At this point it became clear to us that we needed to conduct an in-depth
qualitative study on how previously documented factors, as well as new ones we
might discover, interacted in the daily lives of consumers to affect the development of pressure sores. We reasoned that such a study would give us an in-depth
understanding of not only discrete factors, but also the constellations of factors
that put people at risk of pressure sore development in their daily living contexts.
This knowledge could then be utilized to inform the design of a lifestyle redesign
intervention that we hoped to subsequently test for cost-effectiveness in a
randomized clinical trial.

In 1999, we received a Field Initiated Research Grant from the Natural Institute
of Disability and Rehabilitation Research to undertake such a study. Our inves-
tigative team consisted of a surgeon, a physiatrist, two occupational therapy
practitioners from Rancho Los Amigos National Medical Centre, a consumer, as
well as our USC-based research group. In addition, we established a four-person
consumer board which consulted on the project. The study is enabling us to
uncover the complexity of lifestyle factors that contribute to pressure sore
development as they interact in the lives of people with spinal cord injury. Once
this study is completed, which in essence is serving as a comprehensive and
rigorous needs assessment, we will be positioned to design a lifestyle redesign
intervention that we will test in a proposed randomized clinical trial and cost-
effectiveness study.

14.3.3   Additional treatment populations

Finally, our team has been applying preventive lifestyle redesign interventions with many or all of their signature components (as specified in Table 14.2) to other at-risk populations. One example concerns overweight adults. Thirty-five percent of American adults are overweight, another 26% suffer from obesity, and diabetes is now an epidemic that has increased by nearly 40% in the last decade (Fischman, 2001). To combat these major public health problems we have designed a lifestyle redesign weight-loss programme that stresses healthy eating, healthy living and better regulation of blood sugar levels through natural food intake. Just as the original lifestyle redesign programme stressed healthy daily activities, this new application also emphasizes healthy habit development in at-risk populations. Participants learn about healthy habits of eating and lifestyle and come to understand the relationship between the two. For example, they learn about the

Table 14.2   Similarities and differences between traditional occupational therapy and lifestyle redesign

Similarities
(1)   Focus on occupational storytelling and storymaking. Traditional occupational therapy involves taking occupational histories.
(2)   Content and focus overlaps in certain areas, e.g. safety, transportation.
(3)   Incorporates 'doing' and not just talking.
(4)   Projects used in lifestyle redesign groups can resemble projects used in traditional occupational therapy.
(5)   Group process and one-on-one mode of delivery in both.
(6)   Both rely on activity analysis.

Differences
(1)   Lifestyle redesign incorporates elements based on holistic needs that may not be included in a traditional occupational therapy programme.
(2)   Lifestyle redesign gives more emphasis to the process of planning and enacting a customized routine of health-promoting and meaningful occupation, while traditional occupational therapy may be more narrowly focused on specific tasks a consumer wants to accomplish.
(3)   Lifestyle redesign is focused on a panoramic view of the person in the daily life context. Traditional occupational therapy may place more emphasis on specific deficits due to catastrophic illness or disability.
(4)   Methods of delivery (peer support, didactic presentation, direct experience and personal exploration) are more crystallized and manualized in a lifestyle redesign intervention.
(5)   Lifestyle redesign is usually focused on prevention: traditional occupational therapy is typically focused on remediation and compensation after catastrophic illness or disability.
(6)   Lifestyle redesign stresses conducting needs assessments to tailor interventions to particular target groups and to bracket preconceptions. Traditional occupational therapy may be based more on standardized protocols or textbook content and intervention approaches.
(7)   Lifestyle redesign is highly phenomenological in its approach: traditional occupational therapy may be more focused on performance.

ways in which stress-producing occupations, such as having to write a paper or give a speech, may create a craving for sweets. By the same token, they also learn how to customize their eating so that they have sufficient nutritional support to sustain a healthy routine of living. The end goal is both healthy doing and healthy eating, which must be inextricably linked and sustainable over the life course. We were fortunate that we were able to secure insurance coverage for this programme through the University of Southern California's medical coverage plan.

In part because of the success of the weight-loss programme, USC Care, a corporation that provides health care to USC personnel and citizens throughout Los Angeles, invited us to provide lifestyle redesign consultation in its new executive health programme. In this programme, high-level executives check in to a health care setting for the day and receive a comprehensive physical assessment. As part of the work-up they can elect to have a lifestyle redesign consultation to assist them in developing strategies for living that will optimize their health. The consultation takes into account the interface of typical eating patterns, exercise level, health status, stress, work demands, sources of pleasure, activity patterns, social demands and travel schedules. Following the consultation, the executives are provided with a customized plan for healthy living, including strategies for counteracting potentially health compromising pitfalls that may be part of their typical day or work schedules.

14.4   Preparing occupational therapists to incorporate lifestyle redesign

Due to the widespread applicability of lifestyle redesign, we feel that many therapists, representing different areas of practice, stand to benefit from a deeper awareness of the underlying concepts. Therefore, we have devoted a good deal of attention to training issues. In some cases therapists may profit by integrating component principles into ongoing practice efforts that do not specifically employ a lifestyle redesign programme. In other cases therapists require training in an explicit lifestyle redesign programme, such as the Well Elderly intervention.

Since the beginning of the Well Elderly Study we have focused primarily on training occupational therapists in how to administer lifestyle redesign inter-ventions. Our training has assumed that the therapists have graduated from an accredited occupational therapy education programme and have mastered the essential coursework required for providing services as an occupational therapist. Since not all occupational therapists have had exposure to occupational science, introductions to its major assumptions about occupation are provided initially. These include the centrality of occupation in human existence, the definition of occupation, the effects of occupation on physical and mental health and on life order and routine, and the role that occupation can play in prevention. Other important topics include ways in which occupation can be harnessed to promote transformation, meaning in occupation, dynamic systems theory, occupational science's view of the human as an occupational being, daily 'hassles', adaptation, inventing occupations, the role and structure of ritual, wellness occupations and healthy habits.

Formal courses in lifestyle redesign have been taught both to practitioners, through national and international workshops, and to students through college coursework. It was necessary for us to design various models of lifestyle redesign training because of the different formats used to deliver the information and the recipients' varying knowledge levels. However, in every training session there are three concepts that we have found valuable to cover. These include differentiating traditional occupational therapy from lifestyle redesign, understanding the phenomenological aspects of occupation and integrating new habits into the clients' everyday events of life.

Frequently, students in our lifestyle redesign courses initially have difficulty distinguishing traditional occupational therapy from a lifestyle redesign approach. In order to clarify this difference we have used an exercise in which we ask the class to develop a chart that depicts the similarities and differences between a lifestyle redesign and more traditional occupational therapy approach after they have read the manual. Table 14.2 contains such relevant content. Our experience is that most students will extract similar content for these charts through this exercise, and doing so enables them to better differentiate the two forms of occupational therapy.

Preparing occupational therapists to administer lifestyle redesign treatment is also facilitated by enabling them to fully appreciate the phenomenological aspects of occupation. They must come to fully understand that the same occupation can be experienced differently by different people. We therefore ask our students to do readings in phenomenology. Special emphasis is given to hermeneutic phenomenology (Heidegger, 1927) as well as Gadamer's (1982) concept of communal horizon of understanding and Merleau-Ponty's (1964) notion of embodiment. These readings provoke students to reflect upon the questions listed in Table 14.3.

Exposure to phenomenology enables students to interpret clinical encounters with more depth during their administration of lifestyle redesign groups. They

Table 14.3 Phenomenologically relevant didactic questions

---

(1) How do I experience therapeutic encounters? What are my typical mood states?
(2) What are my patient's moods? What does his or her embodiment convey? What is hidden or concealed?
(3) How do my preconceptions or biases affect my therapeutic encounters?
(4) How can I develop the ability to be open to the horizon of understanding of my patients? How can I develop the skills to build a communal horizon of understanding with my patients?
(5) How is my understanding of myself and my patients embedded in my culture, history and bodily being?
(6) What matters to me? What do I care about most in therapeutic encounters?
(7) How can I best come to understand what matters to my patients and develop interventions that address these issues?

---

come to see that it is crucial for them to consider the ways in which their clients exist in their worlds, try to grasp what matters to them, and be able to read body language during group sessions and individual meetings. In addition, through reading Foucault (1984a, b, c; cited in Rabinow, 1984) they begin to be able to identify the ways in which their clients may be engaged in self-limiting practices. Finally, through exposure to Peloquin's (1993a, b; 1995) writings on therapeutic empathy, they gain a sense of the ways in which we feel they should build relationships with their clients.

As routine and habit seem to be central to the effectiveness of lifestyle redesign programmes, we have also tended to concentrate on imparting these concepts. Typically, students begin by reading articles on habit and routine such as those written by Dewey (1988), Corbin (1999), Clark (2000) and Cutchin (2000). Following this reading, a lecture is given that focuses on: (1) the definition of habits and routines, (2) their functions, (3) their relationship to clinical outcomes in the USC Well Elderly Study, and (4) methods of habit inculcation. In the end, the students grasp the notion that building a life-sustainable, health-promoting daily routine usually requires a reorganization of one's daily activities and habits, and that habits are initially resistant to change. In short, the message is that habit inculcation takes time.

The two student training courses described below exemplify the type of training experiences we have found to be effective.

14.4.1   The 'After Hours' course

The group, comprised of occupational therapy students, named itself 'After Hours'. Food was provided every week and we began the groups with a rapport-building activity in which we asked the group members to name something they had done sometime in their life that they did not think anyone else had done. All of the members of the group were asked to engage in occupational storytelling, as described by Clark (1993) and Clark *et al.* (1996b). Group members were instructed to try to practise the 'art of storytelling' as they recounted their occupational histories, not only in terms of what they had done, but also by highlighting what mattered most in shaping who they had become. Students also practised techniques for evoking stories from one another. Further, as the course progressed, the participants were asked to keep a journal in which they related the topic of the week to their particular life situations and goals. The content of these journals was not shared with the professor or the other students.

For this particular course the following are examples of how specific topics were covered through the group process. The topics and activities discussed below were used to facilitate occupational self-analysis and lifestyle redesign. Through these projects students began to develop a deep understanding of their occupational needs. They, in turn, took part in selecting the topics they felt were most relevant to redesigning their lives.

Inventing rituals

After being exposed to content on the structure and purpose of rituals from an anthropological perspective (Turner, 1988), the students described rituals they had invented to mark particular times in their lives or serve other purposes. These kinds of rituals were distinguished from more customary ones such as birthday parties or religious ceremonies. Among the self-created rituals students described were those that marked occasions such as returning to school, keeping connected with family members, rekindling friendships, dealing with depressive states and celebrating the self. After sharing such experiences, the group created a ritual in which they could all participate and one for a future event in their life.

Daily hassles

Prior to this session the students read about studies that addressed the effects of daily hassles on well-being and mood (Kanner & Feldman, 1991). In this session students shared stories about their daily hassles in terms of people and objects (such as the phone ringing during dinner). The ultimate goal of this group session was to formulate strategies to avoid such hassles or to reframe their thinking about what constitutes a hassle in such a way that they would be experienced as less stressful.

Wellness

For this session, after being exposed to didactic content on the health promoting aspects of occupation, the students were asked to recount their wellness and illness stories. They were then asked to analyse the stories to gain a sense of what constituted healthy pleasures.

The subjective experience of occupation

In order for students to fully grasp the fact that different people engaged in the same occupation can have widely different experiences, the group went for a strenuous hike in the mountains. After the hike each participant described his or her experience to the other group members. The diversity in the subjective reports drove home the fact that what is perceived in one way by one person can be experienced in a dramatically different way by another. This experience primed the participants for a more in-depth understanding of the phenomenology of occupation.

Objects of meaning

In the USC Well Elderly Study and another preliminary study that we conducted on community-dwelling elders (Jackson, 1996) we noted that the elders' homes were filled with objects that they had collected over their lives and that carried deep levels of symbolic meaning. Similarly in the book *Tell Them Who I Am* (Liebow, 1993), which the students were required to read, homeless women tell passionate stories about how their intense need to retain personal household objects drives them to pay for storage lockers even though they are evicted and live on the streets. To sensitise the students to this notion we asked them to bring one precious, one neutral and one disgusting object to the class and describe why they classified each one in its respective category.

Identity and occupation
For this session, students were asked to bring in ten pictures of themselves engaged in occupations that best characterized their sense of self. The objective of the session was for them to depict themselves pictorially as occupational beings so that they, as well as others, could better grasp their essence. During the session they arranged the pictures in a manner that would allow them to best express their occupational story (i.e. chapters in life, montage of pictures, categories of work, rest and play). This was followed by group discussions about who they are and why they chose to tell their story in a particular way.

14.4.2   Lifestyle redesign course

In some lifestyle redesign courses we have taught, we have experimented with alternative methods of having the students undergo occupational self-analyses. These analyses are typically very powerful. For example, in a recent course, students were split into pairs and for six weeks engaged in occupational story-telling, at the end of which they were expected to identify their problematiques defined as those things that threatened them and about which they wanted to do something (see Clark *et al.*, 1996b). Figure 14.1 presents a sample questionnaire that can be used to jump-start the interview process in paired sessions. Following the interview, the students can be asked to reflect upon which questions were the most useful, what kinds of information these questions elicited and what other questions they wish to add.

After midterm the students joined lifestyle redesign groups as participants, with several class members whose identified problematiques were similar to theirs, and each student took his or her turn developing a module on an issue related to the topic of careers. Each person then led the group using his or her self-created module. Using this approach, lifestyle redesign programmes have been developed by students to address problematiques such as 'time management', 'how to say no to the demands of others', and 'how to ensure that you receive credit for the work you do'. These issues are representative of the kinds of problematiques our students identified as troubling them. Using this classroom approach, students not only gained experience in how to interview one another in pairs on issues related to lifestyle redesign, but also in how to construct modules and lead lifestyle redesign groups.

14.5   Conclusion

Occupational science developed over fifteen years ago and over a decade has passed since the day our research group first received funding to initiate the USC Well Elderly Study. Although occupational science was originally conceived as a

1. Detailed history of occupational interests
   - Life by time
   - Life by value
   - How did this shape who you are today?

2. Context
   - Culture
   - Family
   - Work setting
   - Friends
   - Home

3. Activity pattern
   - Circadian rhythms
   - Problem solving
   - Typical weekday
   - Typical weekend
   - Decision making

4. Challenges
   - What currently threatens you?
   - Any obstacles to your goals?
   - Any areas of frustration?
   - Unhappiness?
   - Where do you want to be . . .
     — In 10 years?
     — At the time of your retirement?
     — Before the end of your life?
   - Immortality

5. Values and belief system
   - Overall life philosophy
   - Ideal human being
   - Ethics: right and wrong
     — Good and evil
     — Justice and injustice
   - Religion, spirituality

6. Theories on what makes for a good life
7. Role of occupations in the good life
8. How do you think people in your generation differ from those in your parents' generation?

Figure 14.1　Occupation self-analysis worksheet.

basic science, even as early as 1993 our research group was committed to including within its conceptual boundaries studies that had the potential to demonstrate the effectiveness of occupation based practice. By 1996, Zemke and Clark had described the relationship of occupational therapy to occupational science as follows:

'We are convinced that it would serve occupational therapists and occupational scientists well to think of occupational science as interlinked with practice. Occupational science may, in this sense, be thought of as focusing on the form, function and meaning of human occupation, in all contexts, including the therapeutic context. We believe that the ramifications of a strict partitioning would be egregious, the net effect of which would be fragmentation, division between practitioners and theorists, and the production of poorer or irrelevant research.' (Zemke & Clark, 1996, p. x)

Today, we conceive occupational science as encompassing basic and applied research. It can be seen that using this definition, the USC Well Elderly Study is a type of occupational science. Not only was the design of the intervention derived from basic qualitative studies of the life adaptations of the elderly, but, in that the randomized clinical trial itself tested the effectiveness of an occupation based treatment, it too is occupational science. It is also a clear-cut example of the way in which occupational science can nurture occupational therapy. The study unquestionably demonstrated the impact preventive occupational therapy can have on elders, highlighted the cost-effectiveness of the approach, and positioned occupational therapists to work in new practice arenas to confront the public health problems of the twenty-first century. Moreover, it has led to hypotheses about the ingredients that rendered the intervention so successful as well as inspired the development of interesting course designs for preparing occupational therapists as lifestyle redesign practitioners.

References

Byrne, D.W. & Salzberg, C.A. (1996). Major risk factors for pressure ulcers in the spinal cord disabled: a literature review. *Spinal Cord, 34*, 255–263.

Christiansen, C. & Lou, J. (2001). Ethical considerations related to evidence-based practice. *American Journal of Occupational Therapy, 55* (3), 345–349.

Clark, F. (1993). Occupation embedded in a real life: interweaving occupational science and occupational therapy. *American Journal of Occupational Therapy, 47* (12), 1069.

Clark, F. (2000). The concepts of habit and routine: a preliminary theoretical synthesis. *The Occupational Therapy Journal of Research, 20*, 123–137.

Clark, F., Azen, S.P., Carlson, M., Mandel, D., LaBree, L., Hay, J., Zemke, R., Jackson, J. & Lipson, L. (2001). Embedding health-promoting changes into the daily lives of independent-living older adults: long-term follow-up of occupational therapy intervention. *Journal of Gerontology; Psychological Science, 56B* (1), 60–63.

Clark, F., Azen, S.P., Zemke, R., Jackson, J., Carlson, M., Mandel, D., Hay, J., Josephson, K., Cherry, B., Hessel, C., Palmer, J. & Lipson, L. (1997). Occupational therapy for independent-living older adults: a randomized controlled trial. *Journal of the American Medical Association, 278*, 1321–1326.

Clark, F., Carlson, M., Zemke, R., Frank, G., Patterson, K., Larson, B., Rankin-Martinez, A., Hobson, L., Crandell, J., Mandel, D. & Lipson, L. (1996a). Life domains and adaptive strategies of low-income well older adults. *American Journal of Occupational Therapy, 50*, 99–108.

Clark, F., Ennever, B.L. & Richardson, P. (1996b). A grounded theory of techniques for occupational storytelling and occupational storymaking. In: R. Zemke & F. Clark (Eds.), *Occupational Science: the Evolving Discipline* (pp. 339–361). Philadelphia: F.A. Davis.

Corbin, J.M. (1999). The role of habits in everyday life. Abstract of paper presented at 'A Synthesis of Knowledge Regarding the Concept of Habit', a research conference of the American Occupational Therapy Foundation, January Pacific Grove, Calif.

Cutchin, M.P. (2000). Retention of rural physicians: place integration and the triumph of habit. *The Occupational Therapy Journal of Research, 20*, 106–111.

Dewey, J. (1988). *Human Nature and Conduct.* Carbondale, Ill.: Southern Illinois University Press (Original work published 1922).

Fischman, J. (2001, 25 June). Facing Down a Killer Disease. *US News and World Report*, p. 59.

Foucault, M. (1984a). On the genealogy of ethics: an overview of work in progress (from

Michel Foucault: Beyond Stucturalism and Hermeneutics). In: P. Rabinow (Ed.), *The Foucault Reader* (pp. 340–372). New York: Pantheon Books.

Foucault, M. (1984b). Politics and ethics: an interview (C. Porter, Trans). In: P. Rabinow (Ed.), *The Foucault Reader* (pp. 381–390). New York: Pantheon Books.

Foucault, M. (1984c). Polemics, politics, and problemizations: an interview with Michel Foucault (L. Davis, Trans). In P. Rabinow (Ed.), *The Foucault Reader* (pp. 373–380). New York: Pantheon Books.

Gadamer, H. (1982). *Truth and Method* (G. Barden & J. Cumming, Trans.). London: Sheed & Ward.

Hay, J., LaBree, L., Luo, R., Clark, F., Carlson, M., Mandel, D., Zemke, R., Jackson, J. & Azen, S. (2002). Cost-effectiveness of preventive occupational therapy for independent living adults. *Journal of the American Geriatrics Society, 50*, 1381–1388.

Heidegger, M. (1927). *Being and Time*. San Francisco: Harper Collins.

Holm, M.B. (2000). Our mandate for the new millennium: evidence-based practice, 2000 Eleanor Clark Slagle lecture. *American Journal of Occupational Therapy, 52*, 575–585.

Jackson, J. (1996). Living a meaningful existence in old age. In: R. Zemke & F. Clark (Eds), *Occupational Science: the Evolving Discipline* (pp. 339–361). Philadelphia, Phil.: F.A. Davis.

Jackson, J., Carlson, M., Mandel, D., Zemke, R. & Clark, F. (1998). Occupation in lifestyle redesign: the well elderly study occupational therapy programme. *American Journal of Occupational Therapy, 52*, 326–336.

Jackson, J., Kennedy, B.L., Mandel, D., Carlson, M., Cherry, B.J., Fanchiang, S-P., Ding, L., Zemke, R., Azen, S.P., Labree, L. & Clark, F. (2000). Derivation and pilot assessment of a health promotion programme for Mandarin-speaking Chinese older adults. *Aging and Human Development, 50*, 127–149.

Kanner, A.D. & Feldman, S.S. (1991). Control over uplifts and hassles and its relationship to adaptational outcomes. *Journal of Behaviour Medicine, 14*, 187–201.

Law, M. & Baum, C. (1998). Evidence-based occupational therapy. *Canadian Journal of Occupational Therapy, 65*, 131–135.

Liebow, E. (1993). *Tell Them Who I Am: the Lives of Homeless Women*. New York: Penguin Books:

Mandel, D.R., Jackson, J., Zemke, R., Nelson, L. & Clark, F. (1999). *Lifestyle Redesign: Implementing the Well Elderly Programme*. Bethesda: The American Occupational Therapy Association, Inc.

Maynard, F. (1996). Ethical issues in pressure ulcer management. *Topics in Spinal Cord Injury Rehabilitation, 2* (10), 57–63.

Merleau-Ponty, M. (1964). *Phenomenology of Perception* (C. Smith, Trans.). London: Routledge & Kegan Paul. (Original work published in 1945.)

Peloquin, S. (1993a). The depersonalization of patients: a profile gleaned from narratives. *American Journal of Occupational Therapy, 47*, 830–837.

Peloquin, S. (1993b). The patient–therapist relationship: beliefs that shape care. *American Journal of Occupational Therapy, 47*, 935–942.

Peloquin, S. (1995). The fullness of empathy: reflections and illustrations. *American Journal of Occupational Therapy, 49*, 24–31.

Preidt, R. (2002). An ounce of prevention: occupational therapy improves quality of life for seniors. Retrieved 3 October, 2002 from http://www.healthscout.com/template.asp?page=newsdetail&ap=68&id=508713

Rabinow, P. (1984). Introduction. *The Foucault Reader* (pp. 3–29). New York: Pantheon Books.

Sackett, D.L., Rosenberg, W.M., Gray, J.A., Haynes, R.B. & Richardson, W.S. (1996). Evidence-based medicine: what it is and what it isn't. *British Medical Journal, 312,* 71–72.

Slagle, E.C. (1921). *Training aides for mental patients.* Paper presented at the 5th annual meeting of the National Society for the Promotion of Occupational Therapy, Baltimore (October 1921).

Tickle-Degnen, L. (1999). Evidence-based practice forum – organizing, evaluating and using evidence in occupational therapy practice. *American Journal of Occupational Therapy, 53,* 537–539.

Turner, V. (1988). *The Anthropology of Performance.* New York: PAJ Publications.

Wharton, G.W., Milani, J. & Deab, L.S. (1987). Pressure sore profile: cost and management. *Asia Abstracts Digest,* 115–119.

Zemke, R. & Clark, F. (Eds). (1996). *Occupational Science: the Evolving Discipline.* Philadelphia: F. A. Davis.

Chapter 15
Occupation, Population Health and Policy Development

Ann A. Wilcock and Clare Hocking

15.1 Introduction

This chapter examines the concepts of public health and policy development within occupational therapy. Both concepts are topical within current professional literature as well as in broader health care contexts. For occupational therapists the concepts call for extended or new ways of thinking about familiar problems because of their focus on the health of groups of people rather than individuals. Taking a population health focus results in occupational therapists needing to consider how public policies might impact on the occupational lives of individuals as part of social groupings, how that might improve health or, alternatively, lead to increased risks of morbidity. In considering the related issues of population health and policy development the chapter will cover historical and contemporary perspectives and the World Health Organization's (2001) *International Classification of Functioning, Disability and Health* (ICF), but it will begin by defining and discussing the concepts generally.

Population or public health refers to initiatives that are 'directed to the maintenance and improvement of the health of all the people' (Last, 1987, p. 3). The importance of maintaining and improving population health is extolled by the World Health Organization (WHO), which espouses the view that health is much more than the absence of physical or mental illness because it is also dependent on social well-being (WHO, 1946). National governments around the globe, motivated perhaps by the rising costs of ill-health services, are also concerned with public health. However, within affluent societies particularly, health care has remained largely centred on the reversal of physical or mental illness. That has been in preference to promoting health and well-being to counter ill health occurring in the first place. With such a focus, and despite the WHO's efforts over the last half century, the impact of social factors as a cause of physical and mental illness has been minimized. Equally, the issues of social illness, social health and social well-being have been largely overlooked.

Occupational therapists can capitalize on the dynamic nature of public health as currently viewed by the WHO and many national health authorities. This has not always been the case. As Last (1987, p. 6) explains, public health initiatives and priorities change over time in response to changing perceptions of health and the 'historical and cultural context, available facts about perceived human need, social values and scientific and technical capability to intervene effectively'. Wilcock's (2001, 2002) history of occupation-based therapy describes how it has changed similarly in response to historical and cultural contexts, perceived human needs, social values and scientific and technical capability. Building on this synchronicity, this chapter calls for the urgent adoption and promotion of an occupational perspective of public health. A uniquely occupational perspective on promoting health at a population level would have two aspects. The first is that the relationship between occupation and health would be widely recognized, so that ordinary people could appreciate the health impact of their daily occupations and respond accordingly. The second is that public health initiatives would be directed towards ensuring that all people can engage in socially valued, personally meaningful occupations that satisfy needs, enhance capacities and provide opportunities to realize aspirations and help cope with environmental challenges.

Furthermore, such occupations could promote community cohesion and social integration, and be ecologically sustainable (Wilcock, 1998). In emphasizing that all people should be able to access ways to optimize their health through occupation, the vision espoused in this chapter is founded on the notion of occupational justice. Closely aligned to the concept of social justice, occupational justice is about 'recognizing and providing for the occupational needs of individuals and communities as part of a fair and empowering society' (Wilcock & Townsend, 2000, p. 84). It is a justice of difference in that it recognizes that both individuals and communities have different occupational needs and different occupational capacities.

Public health initiatives are incomplete if supporting policy development does not adequately consider the impact of occupation on health and ill health. This means it is essential that policy planners at many levels recognize the occupational nature and needs of people, as well as those of national safety and economics, for example. The thrust of this chapter is to suggest a direction for an occupationally based vision of public health and policy development, whereby all people have access to a range and balance of occupations that support optimal health and well-being.

Developing, promoting and taking action towards an occupational perspective of health at a public policy level could be occupational therapy's unique contribution to public health. This chapter, therefore, explores the actual and potential role of occupational therapists within the public sphere, in the promotion of population health and the public policies that might support it. The discussion begins with an historical perspective of occupational health, and then considers contemporary developments that support such a perspective. Finally, strategic actions and directions for occupational therapists are considered.

15.2   Occupational perspectives on public health from the past

Until the twentieth century, prevention of illness was regarded as equally important as curative medicine. In some ways, that was because the lack of physiological and technical understanding at that time resulted in disability and death being ever-present concerns. The *Regimen Sanitatis* is an enduring example of advice for the maintenance of good health. Emanating from the time of Hippocrates, the six rules that made up the *Regimen* addressed all aspects of living (Paynell, cited in Croke, 1830). They were actively promulgated until the nineteenth century, and provided the basis for both preventive and curative medicine. The *Regimen* informed the medical fraternity through learned texts, the rulers and the rich through verses written specifically for them, and the illiterate population at large through verse that could be easily recalled. Health care was not separated from other aspects of life, and people in almost every walk of life acted as their own physicians and occupational therapists.

One of the six rules is of particular interest to occupational therapists because it concerns the continuum of occupation that covers rest, action, motion and exercise. Stories and advice about balancing one's motion and rest, derived directly from this rule, abound in the historical literature. One example is Ramazzini's (1705) classical text *Treatise of the Diseases of Tradesmen*, which describes how particular trades influence people's health. Ramazzini, a physician, directed some of his advice about how to avoid illness to professors of learning. For them, his recommendations prescribed not only when was the best time for them to work, but also how work should be integrated with food, physical exercise and sleep. He advised that they 'ought therefore to pursue the Study of Wisdom with moderation and Conduct, and not to be so eager upon Improvement of their Mind, as to neglect the Body: they ought to keep an even balance' (p. 273).

Historical sources also provide examples of the interplay between political events and policies and the rise and resolution of public health needs. Wilcock (2001), for example, has chronicled the establishment of Bridewell Hospital for the occupationally deprived and depraved in the sixteenth century. Known as a House of Occupations, Bridewell Hospital arose because of the massive social ill health that followed the closure of monasteries in England. This occurred because King Henry VIII wanted to marry Anne Boleyn. He forsook the Church of Rome when permission to dissolve his marriage to Catherine of Aragon (his first wife) was not forthcoming, and at this time the monasteries were dissolved. For centuries monasteries had provided the venue for public health and social services for the majority of people experiencing mental, physical and social disorders. Their closure resulted in loss of home, work, purpose and meaning for most of those who provided or received these services, and a subsequent increase of unhealthy occupations and environments. The consequent recognition of the social nature of health by concerned citizens of London led to their supplication of Edward VI for the Palace of Bridewell as premises in which to train the socially disadvantaged in purposeful occupations.

Using a history of ideas approach to uncover and interpret examples such as these, Wilcock (1998) revealed that occupation has always been a central, but often silent phenomenon in the maintenance of health. She also found that, from time to time, occupation had also been recognized as having a contribution within curative as well as preventive frameworks. However, much of this occupational perspective had been lost by the time occupational therapy made its debut early in the twentieth century. That timing accounts, to some extent, for the current focus of occupational therapy within medical, ill-health and disability services rather than in population and health promoting initiatives. For, despite their knowledge of the health giving and curative properties of occupation, occupational therapists have largely been employed within curative medicine and not population health. Gradually their domain of concern has come to be linked with adaptation to overcome disability, based on Western values of independence and autonomy. An almost unquestioned acceptance of this has meant that other aspects of occupation for health appear beyond the profession's domain of concern.

15.3   Contemporary occupational perspectives on public health

Over the last few decades, as an occupational view of health has once again begun to be developed and espoused, adherence to the medical model has been challenged. A potent example of this is the 13-year population study that found that decreased mortality rates of elders were linked with wide ranging occupations, and not only those of physical exercise (Glass *et al.*, 1999). Similarly, occupation focused preventive health programmes that address lifestyle issues of the elderly population have been shown to provide significant health, function and quality of life benefits (Clark *et al.*, 1997).

Despite the growing evidence of the health benefits of occupation, occupational therapy's present day literature is still based mainly upon medical categories and interests. Population and social health is largely ignored. Additionally, because of their long subservience to medicine, occupational therapists have not sought to be politically critical from their own perspective. Mostly, they have relied on a belief that the profession's worth would be clear within the public arena, to fellow health workers and to governments without ongoing explanation. That belief has proved to be naive, as occupational therapists are frequently heard to bemoan a lack of understanding of their role and potential. Even so they still fail to challenge policies, systems or managers of services who restrict occupational therapists' contribution to the most obvious so that it no longer fits their purpose or explanation of health. This occurs to such an extent that occupational therapists' roles often become so reduced and particular that it can be questioned whether a university level education is required.

As Last (1987) noted, population health initiatives change according to historical and cultural contexts. A recent and, we believe, significant change in how health is viewed internationally has been signalled by the World Health Organization's (2001) *International Classification of Functioning, Disability and Health*

(ICF). This development has the potential to provide an impetus for the adoption of a public health focus within occupational therapy as it recognizes the health outcomes of people's participation, or lack of participation, in occupation. Like occupational therapy, the ICF addresses people's capacity to engage in activities, their actual participation and the ways their environment inhibits and supports that. Furthermore, it encompasses self-care, work and leisure occupations as well as domestic, educational, community and civic occupations, such as casting a vote, along with skills such as learning and applying knowledge, self-organization, communication and mobility. From an occupational therapy perspective, here, at the highest level, is an occupational view of health.

Within the ICF, participation is conceptualized in relation to health conditions (ill health or impairment), body functions and structures, and environmental and personal factors, as pictured in Figure 15.1. and defined in Table 15.1. People's functioning is represented at two levels: at the level of body structures and functions, and at an occupational level of what the person is capable of doing (activities) and what they actually do in their current environment (participation). As the developers of the ICF identify, there is not necessarily a linear progression from impairment of body functions and structures to limitations or problems in participation in activity. That is, ill health or impairment are understood to affect body structures and functions, to sometimes but not always result in activity limitations, and to sometimes but not always affect participation. For example, someone who is HIV-positive may have no activity limitation, but have markedly reduced opportunities to participate in work or relationships because of stigma. Personal factors, such as an individual's lifestyle, and physical, social and attitudinal aspects of the environment also influence people's participation in occupation, but again the relationships are not necessarily linear. Rather, the

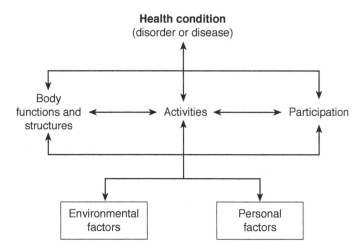

Figure 15.1 Interactions between the components of the ICF. Reprinted with permission from World Health Organization (2001). *International Classification of Functioning, Disability and Health*. Geneva: WHO.

Table 15.1　Definitions of ICF terminology

ICF terminology	Definition
Health conditions	Disease, disorder, injury
Body functions and structures	Physiological and psychological functions and anatomical parts of the body
Activities	A person's capacity to execute occupations (with or without assistive devices or assistance), what the person could do in an envirionment with no barriers to performance
Participation	A person's actual performance of occupations in his or her current environment, including problems the person experiences due to environmental barriers
Environmental factors	Physical, social and attitudinal environment within which people live their lives, which can act as barriers to or facilitators of participation
Personal factors	Aspects of the person not related to their health condition, including gender, race, age, lifestyle, habits, coping style, education, social background, previous experiences, psychological assets, behaviour patterns etc.

interrelationships between all of the factors that influence people's participation in occupation are multiple and complex.

From a public health perspective, perhaps the most important thing to notice about all of the interactions between the components of the ICF is that they operate in both directions. Not only do ill health or impairment affect what occupations people are capable of doing (activities) and actually do (participation), but conversely, participation and activities can affect body structures and functions, and health condition. This, of course, is the premise on which occupational therapy is founded. In addition, when we acknowledge that personal factors, such as habits and lifestyle, affect participation, we can equally expect that people's participation in occupation may bring about change in their personal factors. An example might be people who identify a need to do more of the occupations that provide a sense of competence and subsequently change their lifestyle to accommodate them. Similarly, while the negative relationship between environmental barriers, such as the stigma of having a mental illness, and participation in valued occupations, such as work, are well known, the ICF also provides for influence in the other direction. An example might be employers and co-workers participating in an educational programme designed to reduce stigma by examining the misconceptions on which it is based. The long-term outcome at a societal level might be a higher rate of employment amongst people with a history of mental illness, or those people reporting a higher level of acceptance within the work place. A programme such as this, designed to increase work place participation of a disadvantaged group, both fits the process of enabling occupation described by the Canadian Occupational Therapy Association (Townsend, 1997) and provides an example of action for occupational justice.

15.4   Promoting public health with the ICF

Three key features of the ICF further signal its potential as a tool that occupational therapists might use to develop and promote an occupationally focused perspective of public health. These features relate to the fact that it applies to everybody, its potential to be used as a research tool and its intended usefulness as a social policy or educational tool.

First, as mentioned, the ICF applies not just to those who have a disability but to everyone. The ICF is a description of health and health related states, not merely a catalogue of impairments or ways that health conditions disable people. This means that the ICF could be utilized in a public health context for purposes such as:

- Measuring the incidence of developing a health condition due to participation in high-risk occupations, such as the proportion of people who use a computer who develop symptoms of eyestrain or fruit pickers who develop occupational overuse syndromes.
- Evaluating the effectiveness of health promotion programmes for at-risk groups, such as back care education for mothers of young children or an after school programme for youths at risk of being expelled from school.
- Evaluating the effectiveness of policies to rebalance the effects of economic practices that lead to some sectors of society experiencing stress from overwork, whilst others experience stress from boredom resulting from underwork.
- Monitoring the impact of public health campaigns to promote healthy lifestyles, such as measuring changes in participation in physically demanding occupations at sufficient intensity, duration and frequency to improve cardiovascular health.
- Monitoring the impact of public health campaigns to reduce the stigma associated with mental illness.

Second, the WHO (2001, p. 5) developed the ICF with the explicit intention that it be used as a tool to 'provide a scientific basis for understanding and studying health and health-related states, outcomes and determinants'. Its usefulness to occupational therapists lies in its detailed categorization of aspects of participation in occupation. The WHO's vision is that the ICF be used as a research tool to measure quality of life or environmental factors that influence participation. Our contention is that because of its relevance to quality of life, the ICF can provide occupational therapists working in population health and policy development with a strong argument for research into the relationship between occupation and health, as well as the occupational determinants of health. Such research would provide an evidence base for working in populations with physical, mental or social ill-health concerns. For example, first year occupational therapy students at Deakin University in Australia set about finding evidence related to occupational alienation, deprivation and adaptation within population groups in and around the industrial city of Geelong, Victoria. They found evidence supporting the need for occupational intervention with diverse groups such as single teenage mothers, socially isolated elders and communities with high unemployment.

Third, the WHO (2001, p. 5) envisages that the ICF be used as a social policy tool for, amongst other things, 'policy design and implementation'. The initial challenge for occupational therapists is to identify the occupational component of public health issues, and to envisage public health policies that could address them. One scenario might be that occupational therapists, alert to the health consequences of occupational deprivation, develop guidelines for participation in occupation for at-risk groups: be they prisoners, people in long-term care or people resident in refugee camps. Another scenario might be directing attention to the correlations between youth unemployment, crime, homelessness and poor health, and advising on the development of policies targeting community-based alternatives to work. Such policies would need to address how to provide the health benefits of work, such as exercising capacities, developing relationships, having a daily routine and so on, while still providing incentives to join the workforce should the opportunity arise.

15.5   The ICF and occupational therapy

At the 2002 World Federation of Occupational Therapists (WFOT) Congress, the ICF was used to provide a conceptual framework to organize the programme content and sequence. This gave the ICF prominence as a potential direction for national associations in the 54 member countries that WFOT represents. The ICF has also been adopted in the American Occupational Therapy Association's (2002) *Occupational Therapy Practice Framework: Domain and Process* because it is seen as providing a language and terminology that reflects current occupational therapy knowledge.

Also in 2002, the British College of Occupational Therapists (COT) developed a strategy document with the ICF recognized as a domain of concern for occupational therapy. A diagram (Figure 15.2) encapsulating the COT strategy places the ICF's model centrally, but extends it to emphasize population health and well-being. It highlights how that is dependent on a greater understanding of the ways health is maintained and increased through engagement in occupation, and a commitment to ensuring the provision and enactment of occupationally just policies. This diagram suggests that evidence is required from diverse communities and population groups, along with the perspectives of clients who have been the recipients of occupational therapy. The COT strategy is inclusive in that it recognizes that occupational dysfunction or ill health is not confined to those who have medically defined illness or disability, and that occupational health and well-being is a right of all people and an appropriate responsibility for occupational therapists to assume.

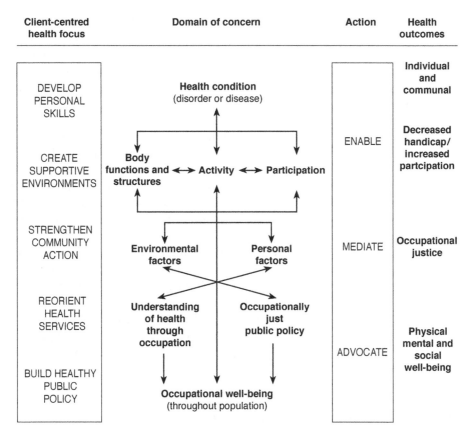

Figure 15.2 ICF set within the *Ottawa Charter for Health Promotion*. Reprinted with permission from the College of Occupational Therapists (2002). *The Response of the Council of the College of Occupational Therapists to 'From Interface to Integration: A Strategy for Modernising Occupational Therapy Services in Local Health and Social Care Communities'*. London: College of Occupational Therapists.

Within the COT strategy the depiction of the extended ICF view is encased in the wider population health vision promulgated in the WHO's (1986) *Ottawa Charter for Health Promotion* (OCHP). The OCHP, while recognized as a classic document of its era, remains current and appropriate in the new millennium. It argues for a health focus that aims, not only towards personal skill development, but also towards the creation of supportive environments, the strengthening of community action and the building of healthy public policy. It places these alongside the call for the reorientation of all health professionals towards the pursuit of health as well as the remediation of illness.

Both the strategic action approaches of the COT and occupational therapy's client centred enabling rhetoric are compatible with the focus of the OCHP. So, too, is the COT strategy that recommends occupational therapists should act as mediators and advocates on behalf of disadvantaged communities and population groups. To be effective in those roles, occupational therapists will need to take a more active role than has traditionally been the case within management, social planning and political levels. This change in political activism may require change in future educational programmes, along with an extended vision of the knowledge and research that informs occupational therapy. The multi-directional and multidisciplinary nature of occupational science is of particular use in these projected circumstances.

The COT strategy is focused towards four major occupation-for-health outcomes for individuals and communities. They are a decrease in handicap; an increase in participation; the creation of environments and policies that are occupationally just; and an increased population experience of social, physical and mental health and well-being. These outcomes are shown in Figure 15.2 to result from the client centred focus, the domain of the profession's concern and the actions taken.

Strategies such as that of the COT provide an impetus for occupational therapists to recognize a wider vision of their role in health care. This vision might build upon evidence from many fields, including historical initiatives of an occupation for health nature such as the public lobbying that led to the establishment of Bridewell Hospital. Researching and enabling similar initiatives in the present day, or in the future when social change or political will disrupt people's need for relevant, balanced and health giving occupation, could be part of a wider vision towards occupationally focused practice.

15.6   Recommendations and conclusion

Given that the relationship between occupation and health remains largely unrecognized, it is not enough for occupational therapists or scientists to engage in public health initiatives or health promotion as they are currently envisaged. Instead, they must bring to population health and policy development their distinct view of people as occupational beings. They must analyse population health research and practice from that perspective, challenging research and initiatives when appropriate, and advocating different research, policies and interventions. Others have recognized such a role. The American psychiatrist, Bockoven (1972, p. 219) for example, considered that occupational therapists had 'a body of moral perspectives and occupational lore of unique value to society' that was relevant to more than a 'service solely for sick people'. He argued that to make use of those perspectives and values was of 'more central importance to future human development than could possibly be claimed by any existing scientific specialty'.

Although some occupational therapy practitioners, educators and leaders in the field have journeyed in this direction from time to time, it remains largely unexplored and uncharted. Its way forward is dependent on research, exploration and initiatives that have a closeness of fit with current population health ideals and policies. These need not, however, replicate the way forward taken by other public health practitioners. Rather they should offer new perspectives, new ways of knowing, and responsive, enabling ways of doing, advocating and mediating. Wide ranging research methods may be used, in addition to the broad based epidemiological methods that tend to be favoured in public health at the moment. Whilst these are vitally important in establishing occupation as a requirement for health in a global sense, many other tools of exploration may be useful to provide direction and detail. Histories of ideas can be useful to view already known facts from new directions; qualitative methods can explore deeper meanings for particular target groups; narrative can suggest avenues beyond the most obvious; and critical action research can involve communities in facilitating social change through self-reflective inquiry and raising levels of consciousness about issues of occupational justice, social health and hegemony. Whatever the method of exploration, an understanding of individual health and well-being through occupation is dependent on an understanding of 'occupation for health' at a population level, and on the development of occupationally healthy and just public policy.

References

American Occupational Therapy Association (2002). Occupational therapy practice framework: domain and process. *American Journal of Occupational Therapy, 56* (6), 609–649.

Bockoven, J.S. (1972). *Moral Treatment in Community Mental Health.* New York, NY: Springer Publishing Co.

Clark, F., Azen, S., Zemke, R., Jackson, J., Carlson, M., Mandel, D., Hay, J., Josephson, K., Cherry, B., Hessel, C., Palmer, J. & Lipson, L. (1997). Occupational therapy for independent-living older adults. *Journal of the American Medical Association, 278* (16), 1321–1326.

College of Occupational Therapists (2002). *The Response of the Council of the College of Occupational Therapists to 'From Interface to Integration: a Strategy for Modernizing Occupational Therapy Services in Local Health and Social Care Communities'.* London: College of Occupational Therapists.

Croke, A. (1830). *Regimen Sanitatis Salernitanum: A poem on the preservation of health in rhyming Latin verse addressed by the School of Salerno to Robert of Normandy, Son of William the Conqueror, with an ancient translation: And an introduction and notes by Sir Alexandra Croke.* Oxford: A.A. Talboys.

Glass, T., De Leon, C., Marottoli, R. & Berkman, L. (1999). Population based study of social and productive activities as predictors of survival among elderly Americans. *British Medical Journal, 319,* 478–483.

Last, J.M. (1987). *Public Health and Preventive Medicine.* Connecticut: Appleton & Lange.

Ramazzini, B. (1705). *A Treatise of the Diseases of Tradesmen, shewing the various influence of particular trades upon the state of health; with the best methods to avoid or correct it, and useful hints proper to be minded in regulating the cure of all diseases incident to tradesmen.* London: Printed for Andrew Bell, Ralph Smith, Danial Midwinter, Will. Hawes, Will. Davies, Geo. Straghan, Bern. Linot, Ja. Round and Jeff Wale.

Townsend, E. (Ed.). (1997). *Enabling Occupation: an Occupational Therapy Perspective.* Ottawa: Canadian Association of Occupational Therapists.

Wilcock, A.A. (1998). *An Occupational Perspective of Health*. Thorofare, NJ: Slack.

Wilcock, A.A. (2001). *Occupation for Health: a Journey from Self Health to Prescription*. London: British Association and College of Occupational Therapists.

Wilcock, A.A. (2002). *Occupation for Health: a Journey from Prescription to Self Health*. London: British Association and College of Occupational Therapists.

Wilcock, A. & Townsend, E. (2000). Occupational terminology interactive dialogue: occupational justice. *Journal of Occupational Science, 7* (2), 84–86.

World Health Organization (1946). *Preamble to the Constitution of the World Health Organization as adopted by the International Health Conference, New York, 19–22* June 1946; signed on 22 July 1946 by the representatives of 61 States (Official Records of the World Health Organization, no. 2, p. 100) and entered into force on 7 April 1948. Geneva: WHO.

World Health Organization (1986). *Ottawa Charter for Health Promotion*. Geneva: WHO.

World Health Organization (2001). *International Classification of Functioning, Disability and Health*. Geneva: WHO.

Index

CPSIA information can be obtained at www.ICGtesting.com
Printed in the USA
LVOW03s0117210414

382374LV00004B/2/P